Dear Tony

Please read

Antoinette Anthony-
Pulán

The Never Ending Journey

Living with Brain Injury

Antoinette Anthony-Pillai

instant
apostle

First published in Great Britain in 2012

Instant Apostle
The Hub
3-5 Rickmansworth Road
Watford
Herts
WD18 OGX

British Library Cataloguing-in-Publication Data

A catalogue record for this book is available from the British Library

This book and all other Instant Apostle books are available from Instant Apostle:

Website: www.instantapostle.com
E-mail: info@instantapostle.com

ISBN 978-0-9559135-6-3

Printed in Great Britain

Instant Apostle is a new way of getting ideas flowing, between followers of Jesus, and between those who would like to know more about His Kingdom.

It's not just about books and it's not about a one way information flow. It's about building a community where ideas are exchanged. Ideas will be expressed at an appropriate length. Some will take the form of books. But in many cases ideas can be expressed more briefly than in a book. Short books, or pamphlets, will be an important part of what we provide. As with pamphlets of old, these are likely to be opinionated, and produced quickly so that the community can discuss them.

Well-known authors are welcome, but we also welcome new writers. We are looking for prophetic voices, authentic and original ideas, produced at any length; quick and relevant, insightful and opinionated. And as the name implies, these will be released very quickly, either as Kindle books or printed texts or both.

Join the community. Get reading, get writing and get discussing!

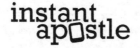

Table of Contents

Acknowledgements

It is a common problem that we never say thank you enough, yet I know that without the help of all the health professionals and my family over these many years my life would be not be what it is today. I have met so many people in my day-to-day life who have treated me with kindness and have tried hard to understand my problems as best they can, and again I am grateful for this. However, I would like to say some particular thank yous.

Thank you to my parents and sister. I love you very much and I know you have suffered and rejoiced with me at every stage on this long journey.

Thank you to all my friends before and friends after my injury.

Thank you to all the people who prayed for me and continue to pray for me, especially Pastor Colin Dye, Pastor William Atkinson and the congregation of Kensington Temple.

Thank you to Suzanna Hoskins for her helpful advice and comments and to Wendy Toole for making sure the sentences on the page were the same as those in my head.

A big thank you to Dr Sherrie Baehr for inspiring and encouraging me to write about what happened to me.

And finally I would like to acknowledge and thank Christ my Lord for saving me both physically and spiritually.

Author's note

My name is Antoinette. I was born in 1973 in Sri Lanka in the beautiful harbour town of Trincomalee. I moved to England in 1977 and have lived in Watford, Hertfordshire, for the last 25 years.

On 25th February 1995 I suffered hypoxic brain damage as a result of a severe allergic reaction to the anaesthetic drugs I was given for a routine tonsil operation. I was a medical student at the time, and the accident happened in the medical school where I was training.

It is more than ten years since my accident; the journey has been long, and it is not over yet. I have decided to write my story for a number of reasons: partly for me – I have always been an achiever and to see my work in print will be the ultimate achievement, and also the process of writing has been therapy for me; partly for my family, as an insight into my life and a record of the last decade of our lives; and partly for all the other brain injury sufferers and their carers. To this end, I hope you like the fact that the book is not too long!

When I wrote the first draft of this book, it was very different from what it is today. My goals were the same, but my account was a positive, breezy look at my life, very much coloured by the fact that I am psychologically and emotionally in a good place at the moment. A few of my friends did say it needed more of me in it. My family wanted me to write down my feelings – this has not been an easy task. My memory of the events and how I understood what had happened to me are very sketchy.

I never was one to keep a diary. I have been asked to keep a notebook and pen in my bag from nearly day one since my accident, but with the best will in the world – and I cannot say how hard I have tried – they are never both in the same place at the same time even when I do remember I should use them. So I finally decided to do what most people with head injury have to do: to rely on the help of my family. They have filled in many of the missing pieces, drawn out of me my emotions and helped me put together a coherent, readable piece of work. I have included many of their reflections and feelings of the past decade of their lives. This is still my story, but their close involvement in it is not such a bad thing, as for many brain-injured people it is not only them who suffer but their families too, and very often it is the families who are left to pick up the pieces.

I know my story is unique – coloured by who I was before the accident, the type of injury I had, the family I am in and many other factors. But I also know that my experiences are not unique, or even uncommon; some have even gone so far as to say that they reflect loss of identity and role, whatever the cause. I hope my story resonates with you, whether you have suffered a brain injury yourself or care for someone who has. I hope this book helps you to understand your dark moments and losses, but also the hope and joy of realising that we are still alive and, boy, do we have a story to tell!

Foreword by Professor Michael Oddy

There is something terribly uplifting about working with people who have had brain injuries. There is a paradox that an injury to the part of us most closely associated with our humanity somehow often reveals the most human qualities and strengths. When a serious brain injury occurs, the individual affected and those around them have to dramatically readjust their view of themselves and indeed of the world in general. Antoinette's story is a familiar yet poignant example of how people negotiate this difficult path, in her case from being a medical student at a prestigious medical school with her sights set on specialising (ironically) in neuroscience. The process takes years, and it is this story that Antoinette tells so eloquently and with such a light and humorous touch. Yet she pulls no punches and does not avoid the darker moments of despair that are inevitable along the way. She shows how important it was for her to try to resume her studies, even though it seemed unlikely she would be successful – once again so often an essential part of the process of adjustment. Nor should one assume the story ends at the end of the book. For Antoinette, and others like her, the struggle continues.

I remember Antoinette in the earlier days of her rehabilitation, quietly composed, contemplative and always evincing a sharp intelligence despite the difficulties imposed by her brain injury. She would, I am sure, have been an inspiring doctor. She is instead an inspiring human being. I hope and expect that this book will inspire her readers as well as those fortunate enough to meet her in person.

Professor Michael Oddy
Brain Injury Rehabilitation Trust

Foreword by Dr Sherrie Baehr

In the summer of 2005 I received a call from Dr Michael Oddy asking if I might have time to see Antoinette …

At the time, Antoinette was working at St John's Wood Library and struggling to keep up. She was optimistic despite her difficulties and 100 per cent committed to succeeding. I was immediately struck by her dedication to her job and her desire to achieve.

Unfortunately, despite all her efforts, the efforts of her very supportive family and the efforts of the library to work with her disability, she was unsuccessful. It was very hard for all to understand why a girl who looked so capable, and was so motivated and intelligent, would be unable to maintain a part-time library assistant post. This is the unfortunate plight of those living with a severe brain injury. You look like every one else and in superficial conversations you sound like everyone else. But the reality is that your brain is processing information in a very different way, making even basic tasks very challenging. To the outside world it may appear that the person is lazy or rude or, even worse, doesn't care.

I will never forget Antoinette's dignity and unshakable hope on the day she was let go from the job she had worked so hard to obtain and maintain. However, in the months following Antoinette suffered repeated failures in her quest to obtain further paid work and sadly her mood declined and depression emerged. During this very dark time Antoinette never lost her fighting spirit and she spent months just trying to put one foot in front of the other, coming to terms with the severity of her injury and how it had altered the course of her life.

Fortunately, it was during this time that Antoinette began to contemplate telling her story to others as a means of helping them. I believe that Antoinette has come full circle and that using her ability to help others overcome disability is what she had set out to do when she entered medical school.

Her story is a wonderful testament to the human spirit, and as you read it you can see the blending of her infallible spirit with the abilities she has retained.

This book is truly inspiring, as it cleverly illustrates the 'never-ending journey' for those affected by brain injury.

Dr Sherrie Baehr
Clinical Neuropsychologist
Founder of The Silverlining charity

The Brain Injury Rehabilitation Trust (BIRT) is the leading brain injury rehabilitation charity in the UK. BIRT offers complex care for people requiring special needs support or suffering disabilities resulting from head injury, including traumatic brain injury, stroke and learning disability issues as a consequence of brain damage.
www.thedtgroup.org/brain-injury/

The Silverlining charity mission is to improve the quality of life of those affected by brain injury. Their work aims to engage the brain injured with the wider community in such a way which invigorates, motivates and rehabilitates them so they can rediscover a sense of purpose and add meaning to their lives, as well as educating the public to the plight of those affected.
www.thesilverlining.org.uk

My sister Antoinette by Rosemarie

Antoinette is fifteen months younger than me; people say we are like twins. We look the same, sound pretty similar and had the same course mapped out, with both of us training to be medics – Antoinette because it was her burning desire, me because I couldn't think of anything better to do: we come from a family of medics. Antoinette always had 'fire in her belly', both figuratively and literally. At only three days old she had her first operation to correct a malrotated gut. Even in those early days there were question marks as to whether she would live or die, and whether she had suffered some brain damage.

Like many who suffer ill health in childhood, Antoinette developed an irrepressible fighting spirit. I was very much the boring, sensible, shy elder sister. I admired her so much. Antoinette, as her Texan uncle exclaimed, was 'full of beans'. She was smart, incredibly funny, infinitely cute and would not take no for an answer.

Her stomach operations stopped her doing gymnastics, so instead she ran, played her violin, got into trouble for misbehaving at school and sailed through her exams. But Antoinette also suffered because of her stomach problems, and when she was sick she was really sick. Her bowels would stop working; often she would ride out the crippling cramps, trying to delay the inevitable operation. As a result she would have lost stones in weight and be vomiting incessantly by the time she found herself in hospital again.

I remember how she would creep into my room late at night: 'Rose, my tummy hurts … will you rub my back? I don't want to wake Mum and Dad.' So in my half-sleeping state I would rub her back till she finally vomited or passed a little wind, after which we could both go to sleep again. I really do believe my sister developed an amazing pain tolerance in those dark hours. Even now her descriptions of pain go from 'it hurts' to 'it hurts a lot' to 'it's really bad': unless you know Antoinette, it is all too easy to underestimate what these laconic statements mean.

Antoinette never let her stomach problems affect her dreams; in fact they inspired her to want to become a surgeon, and preferably a paediatric surgeon. The only thing that got in the way sometimes was her overwhelming desire to enjoy life, party and have fun. As our mum said, Antoinette had a slightly wild daredevil streak – before her accident, she had signed up to do a bungee jump. She loved glitter and glamour and the froth of life. She had a real sense that the world was her oyster, and in many ways it was, and still is.

There was a time when I hated remembering Antoinette before the accident, but now I am glad to remember what she was like – not to regret the 'loss' of my sister, but to remind me where my sister came from, and how who she was ties in with who she is today, and how far she has come.

On 25th February 1995 Antoinette asked me to bring her a change of clothes so she could prepare to meet her friends who were coming to visit her on the ward in the afternoon after her tonsillectomy – she might have been undergoing an operation, but that was no reason not to look her best for her visitors.

I arrived at 11.30 am with a bunch of white calla lilies (I had no idea of the connotation lilies had), but she wasn't back from theatre. One of the nurses found me sitting around on her bed and told me and John (my boyfriend) to go and sit in the waiting room. Feeling suitably chastised, we went and sat in a dingy smoke-filled room. Ten minutes later we decided to go and track down a friend of mine who had recently qualified as a medic and was working as a junior doctor. One hour later we returned to the ward, to be reprimanded once again.

'Where did you go off to? We have been looking for you. We asked you to stay in the waiting room.' They took us to a nurses' station that was upstairs in an enclosed gallery, with windows that actually looked down onto the ward and onto Antoinette's empty bed.

'Antoinette did not have the operation.' I instantly remembered that Antoinette was needle-shy, but surely she couldn't have refused just because of that! 'She is in intensive care. We will take you over to see her. Your dad is here and your mum is on her way.'

Dad met us in the corridor. He had one hand in his pocket, and the other still clutched the stems of his upturned bunch of flowers. Tears silently rolled down his face – I had never seen him cry before.

In the weeks that followed, we cleared out her room at halls. Bizarrely, as part of her forthcoming rag week antics she had a grim reaper costume, which was hanging in the corner of her room. I still remember thinking how absolutely exquisite her lecture notes were; she was working towards an intercalated degree in neurophysiology and had studiously brought her books to hospital with her. Everything was on automatic pilot, and I spoke to John about the distinct possibility that I might have to give up medicine to look after Antoinette at home. We had been told that the chances of her being in a persistent vegetative state were high. But more subtly than that, the accident had caused Antoinette and me to shift roles without anyone telling us or asking our permission. From being the quiet, boring sibling in the background, I now became some sort of mouthpiece, updating friends and family. Though Antoinette recovered, her big personality would recede.

On 13th March 1995 Antoinette woke up. It was a true miracle. She was reborn at the age of 21 years and proceeded to go through the phases of growing up in the space of weeks, from childhood to teenage years. It was very odd to watch. I

17

believe that the age at which Antoinette had her accident is one of the most devastating times for anyone to fall ill, and yet by all accounts your twenties and thirties are when you are most likely to have a brain injury, usually through a trauma such as a car accident or a fall. Just when you learn the skills to move friendships on from the level of superficial party-mates to substantial lifelong kinship, just when you are most likely to meet a life partner because of shared interests and goals, just when you are honing life skills, discerning the nuances of social behaviour and developing work skills, you go to sleep and wake with a blistering headache to find you are alone, your friends all gone, and you are trying to learn these skills from a hospital bed.

I have to say I was very bad at reading up about brain injury. I think my mother was right when she said I really didn't believe anything was wrong. I believed that Antoinette was healed – her waking up was an absolute miracle, and she had no sign of physical disability in spite of half an hour or more with little if any oxygen getting to her brain. It had to be a miracle, and by all accounts a complete miracle. Looking back, I know I did Antoinette a big disservice in not really taking on board what had happened. To accept it was not to deny that a miracle had occurred.

Antoinette had changed. She was anxious, she was extremely forgetful, but funnily she remembered most of what she had learnt in those few years at university. Her memory was bad, but I figured she just wasn't trying. She had no confidence in it because everyone kept telling her it was damaged – they needed to stop telling her that, and then she could get on with life again. I loathed the psychology and neurology reports – they were so negative. I felt they would only reinforce her sense of not being able to do anything. Antoinette could and would do anything: she had been through many trials in her young life and come out on top. But the truth was that Antoinette's brain had been damaged, and the quicker I accepted it, the quicker we could all move on.

Having said that, to believe that just because a brain has suffered a major insult there will be no improvement is also wrong. I have seen Antoinette improve year by year. This is mainly because she, and we as her family, have settled into living with the new Antoinette. I really do believe that the cognitive effects of brain injury are probably some of the hardest for family members to deal with; I found it hard in spite of my medical background. I heard a colleague once comment on a family friend with dementia who she felt was probably faking some of her erratic behaviour. 'How come she remembers some things and not others? She knows to behave and not shout when she wants to,' this lady exclaimed suspiciously. 'I really do wonder if she is putting it on sometimes.' I regret to say that in my mind I sometimes accused Antoinette of the same thing. I found the patchy, inconsistent nature of her memory hard to work out. Why doesn't she write things down, why doesn't she concentrate, why does she get so angry? She never listens to us. Someone new comes along and tells her something that we have been telling her for ages and she believes they are wonderful, and then accuses us of not helping her.

So all this looks bleak. But Antoinette's story is not bleak: it is full of hope. All I can say is that head injury is a journey; it is long and it is very hard for the family, but far more so for the individual.

A year ago Antoinette had to have her wisdom teeth taken out. She had four teeth extracted under a local anaesthetic (with full intensive care cover in case she reacted to anything). She was fine. Later that day the pain felt better so she decided to pick up the kittens she had seen in the animal welfare centre. Then the pain came back and she needed our support and listening ear. For the first time in a very long time I looked at my sister with complete admiration – here she was, trying her hardest to just get on with life.

Antoinette is a butterfly. Her life has a gentle, ethereal quality now and she truly is an inspiration. I will never understand what it is like to be her, to see life through her eyes, but over the years my esteem for her has grown and grown as I wonder if I would have the courage to face life head-on as she does. She still makes mistakes, and over the years she has become more aware of how poor her memory is and this hurts her deeply. But thankfully she and we have come to a place where we live in the moment, trying not to fret over a lost past, or to worry what tomorrow holds.

Chapter 1

Those were the days

It is February 1995. I have just enjoyed the Valentine Ball hosted by the medical school's football teams, and I am nursing my hangover as all good medical students do at some stage of their studies! I am excited – I have been given a provisional place to do a neurophysiology BSc degree in the third year of my medical studies in seven months' time.

Maybe I had some spooky insight into what lay in store for me. I was increasingly fascinated by the brain and all its intricate workings. How could this mass of blancmange be so complex, and better than any computer one could imagine, or in the right hands (so to speak) create something as intricate as a computer? I was in awe!

So I was in the middle of my second year, and preparing for the yearly rag week antics in March, the highlight of the medical student's calendar. I was to be the person in charge of flanning. Flanning: a stunt in which a person, be they student or staff, is accosted by a masked custard-pie-wielding hit man for a price, according to how disgusting one wants the pie to be! You could have baked beans or some concoction of pudding and ketchup, depending on your particular grudge or sense of humour. The flan would be splattered in the face of your chosen target during a lecture or practical. So I was flanning manager, and I was responsible for booking the 'assaults' and collecting money for the rag week charity.

Personally I could not have been happier. I was in London. I juggled doing well in my exams with plenty of beer, Friday nights in the college bar and a huge circle of friends. I was a cheerleader for our excellent rugby team, and put my small

21

stature and loud voice to good use as cox for the rowing teams.

My sister complained that at my 21st birthday party the previous October she was the boring one, invited because of fraternal bonds to take photos of the boozy crowd of nearly 200 friends I'd invited for a lock-in at the Marquis of Manfield pub in Paddington. She couldn't understand how anyone could even know 200 people. My sister was studying medicine at the Royal Free Hospital School of Medicine, another small University of London Medical School. The rivalry between the schools was well known, so it was only right that my friends and I paid her a visit one Friday night and plastered her college walls with stickers reminding everyone which was the superior establishment.

Since I was a little girl I had always wanted to do medicine. I had been born with a malrotated gut and volvulus (no, this is not some big petrol-guzzling car – it means my intestine was twisted so that it malfunctioned and was at risk of strangling itself). I had to be driven in the middle of the night from my birthplace in Trincomalee, Sri Lanka, to the capital, Colombo, to have an emergency operation, and by the time I was twelve I had undergone six operations. I remained under the care of Queen Elizabeth's Children's Hospital in Hackney with my stomach problems until I was 16 years old. On top of this I had broken my arm twice – once playing leapfrog at school, once overbalancing on the stairs while carrying too many toys. Oh, and my sister broke my nose by losing her grip while trying to balance me above her head holding just my right leg. I was nothing if not accident prone: the NHS and I were old friends. One of my greatest desires was to become a paediatric surgeon, and I had promised myself as a child to invent a surgical procedure in which a zip was inserted into your tummy so that you could be opened up with ease whenever the surgeons needed a look. In my childish mind I believed that this would obviate the need for needles and drips, which I had become quite phobic about.

I had a natural ability to juggle work and play, but could get side-tracked. In school I nearly had my prefect's badge taken away after being caught using the teachers' tea, coffee and sugar supplies in a food fight in their staff room. In 1988 there were numerous teachers' strikes taking place nationally. My sister was coming up to her GCSEs; the teachers were only giving lessons three days a week, or sometimes less (and ours was one of the better comprehensive schools). My family got worried, and decided that for our A levels we would go to a private school.

My sister only had the summer to get used to the idea and she hated the move, feeling very isolated for the two years she spent at her new alma mater. I had two years to anticipate the change, and could not wait to move from my comprehensive, whose only claim to fame would be churning out the rogue trader Nick Leeson (actually the brother of one of my old school friends), to a posher, more high-class establishment. I also relished the idea of not being compared to my older sister (who would have left by the time I began), though she often complained that she was fed up with being referred to by the staff as 'Antoinette's sister' rather than by her own name. Even though she was older, I seemed to attract the interest.

When it came to medical school application, my first choice was an obvious one. St Mary's had a particular reputation: it was the classic rugger-bugger, beer-swigging, old-school-tie, academically brilliant place. Competition was high, with as many as 40 applicants for each place. I was an all-rounder: my grades were good; I played in the school orchestra, having reached grade eight in violin and piano; I ran cross-country; and I could talk your socks off. I told the interview panel at St Mary's that medicine was my destiny! I had three offers, including an unconditional one from St Andrews, but I loved St Mary's and they loved me.

To miss the entry requirement by just one grade was a bitter blow, and had much to do with my feeling too settled in my private school surroundings and with my new circle of friends. But, as I said, St Mary's seemed to want me. They held my place for a year on condition that I got my chemistry grade up – which I duly did. Though I ran around like any 17-year-old, I also knew my mind and my ambitions. I realised that slipping up on the A levels was my own fault and must not happen again. In the end-of-first-year medical exams I got some of the highest scores in my year, and was shortlisted for the physiology prize.

In the first year I dated the rugby captain and lived in college halls. Like all good student accommodation, my room had its very own luminescent orange and white traffic bollard, which lay wedged between the top of my wardrobe and the ceiling. I was not tall enough or strong enough to get it down and figure out how to turn off its incessant flashing amber light. Each day seemed to be a party. I managed to scrounge meals from the better cooks in my group, or else I would eat at 'Connoisseurs', the local curry house – after all, they did a ten per cent discount for us students. I was a regular there; they knew me by name and they didn't have to bother with giving me a menu – it was always going to be chicken bhuna and rice. I was truly contented, and at last my childhood health problems and unhappiness seemed far behind.

I had experienced being bullied at school because I did not do gymnastics and had to have time off when I was recovering from surgery. I know that part of me tried desperately hard to fit in and be liked, but I was also well aware that you could not make everyone like you. So for those people who didn't like me I developed an attitude of 'well, it's their loss'. Maybe there was and is a bit of arrogance in me, but talking about my feelings is something I never did. I just gritted my teeth and got on with things. I was certainly not one to feel sorry for myself.

One of my family's favourite childhood anecdotes about me probably highlights the kind of ballsy attitude I had been born with. It was 1982 and I was eight years old. We were living in Coventry and were one of a handful of Asian families in the area. We had new neighbours, including a teenage boy who insisted on shouting out racist jibes at my sister and me as we walked to school.

'Oi, Paki. But, but, ding ding,' he would shout, with a little sideways wiggle of his head.

'What does he mean?' I wondered. 'We don't talk like that.'

'I don't know what he's saying – let's just ignore him. He will soon get bored and stop,' said my ten-year-old sister sagely. She stepped up her pace, hands firmly in her pockets, head curled into her shoulders, trying to retreat into the security of her duffle coat like a nervous tortoise.

But ignoring was not my solution. A few days later my mother was approached by this boy's mother.

'Dr Anthony, I have to apologise for my son's behaviour,' she said.

'What behaviour?' my mum enquired.

'Your daughter visited me yesterday. She told me my son had been shouting "Paki" at her. She told me she is not a Paki but is Sri Lankan. She said that my son can call her Sri Lankan, she won't mind, but if he insists on calling her "Paki" she will call him "Pinky". I have told my son he has to come and apologise to you and your family.'

Not only did the boy apologise, but he also became a good friend and guardian, like an elder brother to me.

Since 1986 my stomach problems had settled down, but in the early 1990s I started to develop allergic reactions to medications. Once when I was staying with my family in the States, I took some Tylenol for headache and ended up in casualty, unable to breathe. I was told I was allergic to the paracetamol in the Tylenol capsules. Later I had a similar reaction to aspirin-type drugs. My choice of simple painkillers was non-existent. Thankfully I seemed to have a high pain threshold, probably as a result of my stomach problems, and I seemed to manage any aches and pains just fine with ice packs and heat pads.

In my first year of medical school I got one throat infection after another – probably too much boozy karaoke, some would say. But it was starting to affect my work and my ability to concentrate, especially as I could not take paracetamol or anything else for the pain. I finally decided to have my tonsils taken out. Rag week that year was sometime in March, and I had organised my tonsillectomy operation so that I could do rag week and then have recuperation time before my mid-term exams at the end of March. I needed to pass these exams well if I was going to be allowed to take a year out of medical training to do my neurophysiology degree.

My operation was booked for the morning of 25th February 1995. This is the day when my journey began: a journey I had not signed up to; a journey in which for many years I was a bemused and reluctant follower, led by health professionals and family; a journey from which I could not take my leave or turn back.

Chapter 2

The sky falls in

I know nothing of my time in intensive care. In fact, my memory stops nearly two weeks before I even went into hospital to have my tonsils taken out and restarts in a patchy manner more than three weeks after the accident. Even my family seemed to have little idea what had happened. My operation was booked for nine or ten in the morning. They were only allowed to see me in intensive care at five in the evening – by all accounts the staff were anxious that nothing be said to my family until the head of anaesthetics was available to speak to them. After all, my mother is a doctor, my sister was a medical student and I was a student in their own medical school at the time.

My parents were told that I had had an allergic reaction to one of the anaesthetic agents they had given, and had suffered a cardiac arrest. Three days later, in the early hours of the morning, one of the ICU doctors admitted to my mother and sister that I might have been without oxygen for five minutes or more. My family were devastated. They instantly knew that the chances of permanent brain damage as a result were high, even if I were to wake up. A nurse sought my mother in the corridor and said we needed to get legal advice, as something had gone terribly wrong. Ambulance-chasing lawyers accosted my parents in hospital corridors, presumably on someone's tip-off, to give them their firm's business cards.

Over the years we have had a chance to look at my medical records and piece together the events of that February morning. My allergies had been dutifully recorded by the clerking doctor. However, a delay in theatres meant that my case was moved from one theatre room to another. Here it is unclear whether the new doctors had registered the severity of my allergies. I was given a muscle relaxant, which I reacted to: I slowly turned blue. The buzzer on the oxygen saturation machine was silenced (this is not uncommon) and, probably because of my medium-dark complexion, they didn't notice what was happening. The anaesthetics record shows that it took nearly ten minutes from my developing the reaction to my heart stopping, and all the while the adrenaline needed to effectively treat my allergic reaction was an arm's length away.

Everyone who has read my records believes the ten-minute delay must have been an error in logging. After all, if it were true I really should have died. The only other explanation is the one that I and my family believe: that the log was indeed correct and it was purely a miracle of God that I didn't die. Instead I arrested, and numerous teams worked to try to restart my heart. I had 30 minutes of vigorous chest compressions (I now have a bend in my back as my ribs broke and healed at an angle); my lungs were full of fluid (a reaction to the lack of oxygen – my brain swelled with fluid for the same reason). They shocked me at least 13 times, leaving my chest burned by the electric currents. I was 21 years old, and one of their own medical students. They couldn't let me die. They worked tirelessly and brought me back from the brink. I was in a pathetic state, and to cap it all my tonsils were still in place – I had never made it from the anaesthetic room into the operating theatre.

I stayed on the ventilator for 24 hours. The scan of my brain showed severe cerebral oedema (swelling). As I came off the ventilator I became agitated, pulling at the various tubes that had been placed in my neck, in my arms, in my bladder. I wanted to climb out of bed and was deliriously replaying a party where I had lost my shoes – this provided a scrap of light relief for my exhausted family and a couple of friends who were visiting. A few of my medical school friends decided it would be a good idea to test my responsiveness by calling out the names of different boys in my year and seeing if my heart rate went up. (Though this seems a little funny now, when I heard about it later I was extremely annoyed and told them I wanted nothing more to do with them.) My family stuck pictures of me that were taken the week before the accident above the nurses' station where they recorded my observations; they were desperate that everyone should know that this bundled mess was not me.

My sister says that on the first evening I was in intensive care she had told a friend that one of her greatest senses of possible loss was that she might have no one left who shared her childhood memories. We had moved house a lot in those early years after moving to England, led by where Mum and Dad found work. We obviously had school friends, but they came and went with all our moving around, so in one sense I suppose Rose and I really only had each other. Our childhood had its ups and downs, but my sister and I enjoyed recounting the happier times. Though we were very different personalities, we really had a good relationship. Of course we fought – Rose could be particularly nasty. I remember she used to say, 'Well, if you are going to tell Mum I had better give you something to tell her about,' and then proceed to give me a Chinese burn (no hard feelings, Rose). The idea of not being able to recount her childhood memories to someone and have agreement on how things were made Rose feel these memories were somehow anchorless, invalid and in danger of vanishing altogether.

I remember nothing of those days. Supposedly I developed severe movement disorders, which was either due to my brain being starved of oxygen or a side effect of some of the drugs they were giving me to stop me being so agitated. I had to be nursed on two mattresses on the floor. They tried to feed me with a tube down my nose, but it would move with all my wriggling and the feed went into my lungs instead, giving me pneumonia. Then they tried to feed me by putting the feed straight into a vein in my arm, but again the drip got dislodged and my arm filled with fatty, sugary feed. My skin split under the strain of all that fluid in my tissues and the dreaded MRSA bugs then settled on my skin to grow fat and healthy. I still have the thickly scarred ulcers in homage to my MRSA friends' presence – I am only lucky that my arm didn't fall off!

Recently my sister explained how three or four days after I had been admitted to intensive care she and her friend Kirsten decided to stay the night there with me. Over the weekend my family had all slept on the floor of the seminar room, in which the nurses had kindly laid mattresses. Come Monday the room was in use again and so my family had to move out, which probably wasn't such a bad thing as it forced Mum and Dad to go home and get some proper sleep. My sister had decided to stay and go home in the morning after my parents had returned. A friend of mine had lent her a small CD player and so through the night she played a copy of a Moods CD I had bought a few weeks earlier, and had loved. She says how I would move around the mattresses, my legs getting tangled in the catheter tube that was draining my bladder, my arms flinging out and sometimes hitting my face, and my face involuntarily contorting into grimaces and smiles.

Even though my limbs were constantly moving, my body as a whole was limp, so that if you tried to lift me up I was like a rag doll and my head would flop forwards . Sometimes I would come to rest on Rose's lap and she would stroke my hair, which was wet with sweat from all my exertion. Tunes like 'Goodbye Mr Lawrence', the theme from *Inspector Morse*, Adiemus and Delibes's 'Flower Duet' would be playing in the background. She said it was extremely serene, and extremely sad. I never imagined that when I was in the coma I had been moving around – it came as a real shock when I found out. Rose admitted it was something that as a family they never really spoke about, since it served no purpose to anyone and they were aware that these were memories that all three of them shared but from which I was excluded.

When, after the event, I asked Rose (by then qualified as a doctor) if she was traumatised by my accident, she admitted that for a number of years she found it difficult going to see patients in the intensive care unit, especially at night. The noise of the machines and the half-light took her straight back to my time in intensive care, and she felt like crying, but she would tell herself to get a grip as I had neither died nor had any permanent movement problems. It is only now, more than ten years on, that I am starting to get a glimpse of the trauma my family experienced. After my accident my life had closed in and I became an island; nothing touched me and I couldn't reach out emotionally or touch anyone. I know some of this was a natural defence put up by my brain against the trauma I had suffered, but also my depression and changes in how I perceived my environment meant that I found it difficult to see things from another person's perspective. Things are better now, as my family happily inform me.

My friends descended on the intensive care unit daily and would peer in through the glass in the alarmed doors. My family did their best to keep as many as possible of them away. My parents had made a big mistake when a boy visited who said he was a good friend of mine. Mum and Dad had grown used to my dystonias (abnormal movements), and after a brief warning that I was probably not how he remembered me, they let him in. The next thing they heard was the sound of him throwing the big bunch of flowers in his hand to the floor and then running out sobbing bitterly. Mum and Dad felt awful. After that, most friends were kept away. Instead, the clinical tutor and a couple of my friends did a daily update each morning for my year before lectures started. Many also received counselling.

Friends and family visited from all over the world, and half the Sri Lankan community of southern England came to say hello. My sister started to get angry because of the limits on numbers visiting ICU patients. When visitors came, Rose was always banished to the waiting room and she resented the intrusion, feeling they were coming to gawp or as some self-imposed matter of duty. She told a few of them to go away, which understandably didn't go down too well. Mum felt they should have a chance to see me; they had travelled from far and often came with food and good wishes. I also had a very special visit from the dean of the medical school. He sat with me on the floor. It was his retirement year, and it was clear this was not a good way to finish his time at the medical school. He apparently kissed my cheek and left me a small rose plant.

On 10th March I was moved from St Mary's to the renowned National Hospital for Neurology and Neurosurgery at Queen Square in London – my dystonias were showing no sign of improving in spite of heavy medication. My family were pleased about the move. They needed a change of scene, and their confidence was at a low. To be fair, St Mary's probably felt a little at a loss too, with the streams of people coming to visit, and my family's constant less-than-impressed watchfulness. A scan done on the day I was transferred showed that my brain was still severely swollen.

At Queen Square they decided to stop almost all my medications, and my contortions slowly ceased. However, my limbs became rigid; my arms were flexed, and my hands tightly curled. I had developed a piercing cat-like cry. My skin had become greasy and spotty. My sister says that the day before I woke up there was a story in the news of someone who had been left severely brain damaged (ironically, after an anaesthetic accident similar to mine) and was in a coma that had lasted for many years. He had just won some legal case. Supposedly, I looked just like him.

After 17 days of coma (coma is not always the serene, inactive state that is seen on television), my neurologist at last took the decision that it was time to let my family know that the outlook was grim and I was unlikely to improve. To my family this did not come as surprising news.

That was the day I 'woke up' – good timing, or what?

I awoke to find my hair cut – butchered, as I exclaimed. My thick, black shoulder-length hair had become a matted mess, and I instantly thought that my mother had used her amateur haircutting skills, which had lain dormant since our junior school days, to give me a cut that left me looking like Doc Brown from *Back to the Future*. In fact, it was not her fault at all – this had been a professional job, with my hairdresser pleading that she was trying to do the best she could 'under the circumstances'. I remember my throat feeling sore. It was a sensation I remembered from childhood and I instantly knew it was due to the nasogastric tube they had placed to feed me. My arms were tightly flexed upwards, and my fingers scrunched into a ball. When anyone tried to move or straighten them a ripping pain shot up my arms. It's a pain I could never forget.

My earliest memory of that time is waking up in the National Hospital Intensive Care Unit and the bed I was in. I can sort of remember what I must have seen from my bed. The nurses' station was ahead of the bed but slightly to the right, and the doors to the ICU were directly in front. Around my bed were numerous members of my extended family – relatives who had travelled from California and Toronto were all here in London, as though gathered for a party no one had bothered to tell me about! I later heard that my aunt from Texas, whom I am convinced I saw or at least sensed as being with me, had also been at the hospital, but in fact she had returned home just that morning with only the doctor's grim prediction of my fate in her mind.

Now if you ask my dad, he says the first thing I said in my weakened guttural voice was 'Dad'; but if you ask my mum, she says the first thing I said was 'Mum'! Which is correct? I will never know! But I did identify members of my family, and news travelled fast around the medical school that I had woken up. So my friends lined up to see me. It took a while as you were only allowed two visitors at a time per patient in the ICU.

The rest of my memories are very patchy. I can remember going outside to the quadrangle in Queen Square one sunny spring day, and being pushed in a wheelchair by my sister. I had become very frail in the three weeks I spent in intensive care and had lost some of my coordination and muscle tone, which meant that I was unable to walk for a good few weeks after I had woken up. Rose always smiles as she reminds me how I rested my head on my hand, sighed and exclaimed how beautiful the world was and how pretty my sister's friend Kirsten was, and still is! I was very twee and quite cute, I suppose.

One thing puzzled me, though: I could understand that I had been ill and everyone had been worried about me, so why had my rugby captain boyfriend not visited? My mother explained that we had split up several months earlier and he was no longer my boyfriend. I cried – it was news to me.

Chapter 3

The early years

The experts say that an indicator of the severity of a brain injury is the degree of post-traumatic amnesia (PTA) or loss of memories after the accident, and the degree of retrograde amnesia or loss of memories before the accident. I am told my retrograde amnesia was at least one week, if not more. My memory since the accident is patchy, jumbled and sometimes possibly false – for example, I used to believe that the friend who had run out of the St Mary's intensive care unit later came to visit me in Queen Square one evening, after Rose and Mum had gone home, yet my family would stay well past the end of normal visiting hours, and they inform me that he was so traumatised by the first encounter that he never came back. I don't know, and I suppose it doesn't really matter.

I think it was the day after my dramatic awakening that I was transferred out of the intensive care unit onto a regular ward. Yet again I had the bed right in front of the nurses' station so I had to be on my best behaviour! I recall lying in my bed on Lady Ann Allerton Ward and being chastised by the nurses and my consultant for adopting what was then a very characteristic horizontal position. I was ordered to sit in my delightfully uncomfortable and sweat-inducing PVC hospital chair to try to stay awake, but in those days I could fall sound asleep standing up.

I remember the registrar doing his rounds, asking me how I was and examining me. To my horror, my legs were all stubbly with hair, and I would giggle like an embarrassed Geisha and apologise for their unsightliness. My sister describes how each day for three or more days, rather like in the film *Groundhog Day*, the registrar and I would have the same interaction. He would examine my legs and I would giggle in horror. Finally my sister could stand it no longer and my legs got shaved.

My mum and sister would come every evening to toilet me, bathe me and get me ready for bed. I used to cry as I thanked them for looking after my personal care. I had become very childlike, even telling my mother that I was 16 years old and asking why they had put me in an adult ward. Once I caught a glimpse of myself in the lift mirror as I went down to physiotherapy in my wheelchair. I have always been proud of my appearance and I couldn't believe how much I had changed, and how old I looked – I cried.

In the summer of 1995 plans were made to move me on for further inpatient rehabilitation. I visited the brain injury rehabilitation unit at the Homerton Hospital in London. We were sitting in the waiting room. I sat alone, my family a few feet away. I remember a man walking up to me. He was dressed in a gown; he smiled at me and then pulled his gown open to show off his 'birthday suit' in all its unfettered glory. My mum walked over after the man was moved on, and told me not to get upset and not to worry. I responded, 'Why should I be upset? He is brain-injured, just like me.' Mum said she was very proud of me at that moment. The journey was a waste of time as the Homerton had no female beds, so we had to look elsewhere.

I finally got my placement a little closer to home. I moved from Queen Square to Northwick Park Hospital to receive my NHS provision of three months' brain injury rehabilitation. Just before this happened I had to visit my GP, as it was part of the referral protocol in the era of fund-holding practices. It was only two or three months after my accident. The doctor ventured to give her expert opinion: 'This is all just functional' (in other words, all in my head). 'She needs to realise she is a pretty girl. If she can't do medicine, so what? She could easily get married or work as a checkout girl. It doesn't matter – life goes on.'

My mother was furious at this dismissive analysis of my situation. Maybe the doctor was trying to get a reaction, to rile me out of any self-pity she believed I was wallowing in. What she didn't realise was that my lack of motivation and apathy was so deep that her words had absolutely no impact on me. All she achieved was to show my mother that a medical qualification doesn't mean you understand anything about the effects of brain injury, or even know how to be gentle and kind! Fortunately, she signed my paperwork anyway.

Northwick Park Hospital was one of the medical school's teaching hospitals so I frequently saw some of my old friends, which was a confusing experience. I did enjoy seeing my closer friends, but even then it was clear our lives were moving on along divergent paths, and seeing them reminded me of my losses. At that stage my loss was not being at medical school – funnily, it was not the personality changes and slowness in my thinking, which were apparent to all around but not to me.

Once I had to make a journey into town as part of my rehabilitation. I had to buy my own ticket, get on the tube and find my way to St Mary's. My therapist followed a few yards behind like a furtive private investigator. It was harder work than I had expected. I found it hard to think methodically or to pre-empt what I needed, so I fumbled around for my purse and then forgot to take my ticket. The busy-ness of the platform and the noise confused me and I forgot my train of thought. Thankfully I had a clear list of instructions given to me by my therapist that I held onto tightly. I finally made it to my destination – exhausted and desperate to get back to my bed.

Once I had arrived at the hospital, I was horrified to see an old classmate walking down the road (this really should not have been that unexpected, given that St Mary's was where I was training). I was desperate for him not to see me so I hid behind a pillar. I dreaded that he might ask me questions, such as what was I up to – I just had no answers that I considered worthwhile. I didn't consider what would happen if someone else saw me and asked what I was doing hiding behind a pillar for so long.

I spent three months at Northwick Park hospital. Initially I was in my own room, but then they moved me onto the ward to try to encourage me to interact with other patients. I was soon in charge of purchasing fellow patients' newspapers and magazines. This was a very responsible duty as I had to handle other people's money and property. Now I look back at those days with some degree of fondness, but my family tell me I hated it, which is probably the reason why I cannot remember a single fellow patient. By all accounts I wasn't the compliant patient I remember myself as being. Often when my family visited they would find me lying motionless, staring at the ceiling, arms straight by my sides, fully clothed on the bed like a medieval stone carving atop a sarcophagus. My parents say that I could not understand why I was there and why the psychologists wanted me to do such puerile activities – after all, I was a medical student, and a good one at that. I wanted to leave and just get back to medical school, and my old life.

Along with the other brain-injured patients, I produced the rehabilitation ward's monthly newsletter. In this I proudly boasted about being a medical student in one of the top London medical schools. I explained how I was thrilled to have got into medicine as it had been my childhood dream, and couldn't wait to get back.

It was during that summer that I visited my old church. I suppose that since starting medical school my spiritual life had definitely been on the back burner, but I believed God had cured me of my stomach problems in 1986 and since that time my mum, my sister and I had become born-again Christians and were attending a large church in Notting Hill Gate. When the accident happened one of the first people to come and visit my family was the Revd June Freudenberg. She was in charge of prayer and pastoral care for the sick. She had never met me or my family before, but she visited my family at nearly midnight, travelling alone by public transport to the hospital after her prayer meeting had finished, on the night of my accident. It was an act of selflessness, more than duty; she could have visited in the morning. Maybe she knew none of them would have been sleeping that night. Often in those dark hours companionship is all the more vital. My family were forever grateful, and from that day she became a close family friend.

The senior pastor of the church had visited me at St Mary's, appalled at the state I was in. Now was my first visit back to church in years. As soon as the pastor spotted me in the congregation he excitedly called me on stage so that everyone could rejoice in answered prayer. They anointed my head with oil and prayed for me, and everyone cheered. The congregation of nearly 5,000 people had been mobilised into praying for me, but I was oblivious to all this. I had no idea that these strangers had heard my story and had diligently prayed for me in their homes and at church each Sunday. I had no real understanding of what my story was, so as to be grateful or to acknowledge their concern. My family said I gazed out at the crowd, not a flicker of a smile on my face. I had come back from the dead but was no more than a zombie.

My family were anxious. They, and I think the pastor, knew straight away that it was a mistake to make a spectacle of me. I wasn't angry; I wasn't resentful. I was numb and extremely bemused. I refused to go to church after that. Thankfully, one of the other pastors who had visited me at Northwick Park and had received a sharp dismissal from me was astute enough to tell my family to let me be – not to worry, and just continue to pray for me. It took many months before I could go to church again.

After the numbness came some anger. After all, I had not asked for any of this to happen. My life had already been quite tough, and this just was not fair. But more than that, there was the deep frustration that I just could not concentrate in that throng of people. The hymns I had once enjoyed gave me a headache. I tried to concentrate on the sermon but would just drift off and stare at, or more often through, the rest of the congregation, sometimes wondering if I liked a particular outfit, or captivated by someone's Jimmy Choos. I know church may be like this for some non-brain-injured people, but it was a new experience for me.

I was encouraged by my physiotherapist to exercise. I was set stretches, and a jog around the hospital grounds every day. That certainly increased my stamina. I spent from June to August 1995 in Northwick Park hospital. I was then discharged to go home.

I have little to say about the few months I had at home. In the early weeks after my accident I was loving and childlike, thankful, with tears of joy for all my family's hard work. As the weeks went by I changed to become emotionally blunted, refusing to hug or kiss any of them for months. My mother recounts how when she and I visited a shopping mall, I had asked to sit on the bench while she went round the shops. I said I preferred to just watch the other shoppers. My mother looked on from afar as I just sat with drooped shoulders, staring vacantly into space. She said I looked like an empty shell, all life gone.

My sister tells me about the day she found me sitting watching TV while the frying pan in which she had been cooking bacon or something caught fire. She had misguidedly asked me to keep an eye on it while she popped upstairs. She returned to find the kitchen filled with smoke. She frantically tried to put out the flames while I remained seated on the sofa.

I briefly turned round to see what she was up to then returned to watching the television.

It was clear I could not be left alone so my mother employed a carer to come and look after me during the day and to give me my meals while they were at work. I could sleep for long periods and was emotionally very flat, but it was not pure depression. Motivating myself was simply impossible. I liked (if that is the right word) staring at the television for the hours I was not asleep. Now I am well, the idea of watching daytime television makes me feel sick, and I sometimes think that if you are not ill already then watching daytime television will bring on an illness in you. (The only show I do insist on watching is *Neighbours* – a rather sunny, undemanding soap opera from Australia. As students at St Mary's we would all gather in the common room with our lunch to get our daily fix of the goings on in Ramsay Street. *Neighbours* finished at 1.50 pm, after which it was a quick dash back to college for the two o'clock lecture.) My mother was anxious that too long spent sitting around all day in an unstructured environment would just make me go backwards very quickly, and undo any of the benefit I had received from the rehabilitation.

My family tried to get me out of the house and to meet people. But I had completely lost the art of socialising. I would sit and stare without expression. If people asked me a question, I would reply with a simple 'yes' or 'no', often delivered with all the warmth and friendliness of a barking terrier. Once I was at a barbecue at John's house (John was then my sister's boyfriend and is now my brother-in-law). One of his college friends asked me how I was and what I was doing. Supposedly I told him I was going to do a degree in neurophysiology.

'Oh,' he said. 'Do you like physiology?'

'No,' I snapped back, sounding irritated (although I wasn't). He was more than a little startled, but then decided I must have some kind of off-the-wall sense of humour and giggled. He still reminds my sister of our encounter, even after so many years.

In those early months and years I didn't even know how to modulate my voice, which could be loud, aggressive or irritated without my even realising. Making conversation with me must have been very hard work, and people soon gave up, slowly edging away and finding someone else to talk to. I didn't care, and I couldn't be bothered with going out so resisted making further attempts at social interaction. My sister tried in vain to teach me how to make myself more interesting (now that really *was* a role reversal for the two of us!). She would tell me not to fold my arms, not to look so annoyed, to ask questions back to the person, to smile, to nod, to speak softly – it was all a load of nonsense as far as I was concerned. In my head I looked just as I did when I was at medical school. Why didn't she stop talking, go away and leave me alone?

I didn't see myself as others now saw me. My sister found it really hard to accept how I had changed. Even though I was oblivious to how people responded to me, my sister was all too acutely aware. She would introduce me to her friends, and I think she was really upset if they looked down on me, pitied me or just ignored me. She says she felt like screaming, 'Antoinette was and is better, brighter, smarter, wittier than any of you lot.' Nonetheless, she admits that although she felt hurt by some of her friends' reactions, it did not stop her feeling angry towards me, too, for no longer being the vivacious, talkative sister she had known all her life.

My mother tried desperately to get me more rehabilitation. It had become apparent to her that I worked best in the rehabilitation environment, although I didn't like being there – I tried harder to work with the therapists, and my excuses were less likely to be tolerated when I was surrounded by other brain-injured people. My family were aware that I have always been proud, so in these environments I worked hard not to lose face or to forfeit the admiration of my therapists. I went onto various waiting lists for more rehab but I was low priority, having already received my statutory three months at Northwick Park. My parents were told that the only other option would be care in a long-term residential facility for people with learning disabilities, to teach me social skills and independent living, but the idea of an institutionalised life was too much for my family to contemplate for their once lively, clever daughter.

My mum was right. Even though I needed close supervision, I do not believe I would have survived emotionally or mentally in a care facility. Early on in my recovery my liking for the finer things in life was there, even if I didn't have the energy or motivation to act on my likes and dislikes. My taste – and maybe my snobbishness – hadn't changed. It would also have shattered my relationship with my family, as I know I would have felt that they had abandoned me. I felt this to a degree anyway. We needed more time to see what my optimal recovery would be before taking such a major decision about long-term care. The only options were to look at the private sector, or abroad to the United States.

Chapter 4

A family affair

I know I am very fortunate to have a loving family, and it is interesting to see how they responded to my brain injury in different ways. Looking back, it is clear it was not only I who was grieving. We all were – all four of us spinning in our own orbits, trying to come to terms with the changes my accident had inflicted on our lives. My father, who is a civil engineer by background and therefore the only non-medic in my family, simply believed a positive attitude was all that was needed.

We had a special relationship. We looked alike, and I was definitely Daddy's girl. He had left home when he was 20 years old and spent a decade studying in Russia, Germany and Japan. He had many childlike qualities and attitudes. We would see pictures of him as a young man sporting an Omar Sharif 'tache and hanging out with his friends from the ballet companies in Russia and Japan. He loved languages and the arts. With time he lost his hair and became the spitting image of Yul Brynner, and in fact my dad was very similar to the King of Siam in *The King and I*, to the point that my sister and I would invariably cry when watching the film, and not just at the end. When we were children I remember him trying to make us cringe with embarrassment by breaking into song while we were out shopping. He played magic tricks and made really awful jokes. He enjoyed his martial arts, especially judo, and he did not 'do' sickness at all; in fact he avoided hospitals.

Like me, he was not one to express his emotions and feelings – these were not even words in his vocabulary. My mother said that seeing me in the intensive care unit at St

Mary's had a bad effect on him, but one that he never spoke about to us. I knew he admired my wild streak, and although he was not impressed when he got phone calls from me to say that I was OK and that I was in Dublin on a charity dash, not in Paddington as my family had thought, I knew there was a part of him that was smiling and saying proudly, 'That's my girl!'

My sister also seemed to be hoping I would just be OK. I wanted to be OK and believed I was, and she believed along with me. We both fought my mum's realism, mistaking it for negativism. But Rose now admits that her denial actually meant she reacted quite harshly to me, annoyed at what she perceived to be my laziness or rudeness.

Since the accident happened my family had sought legal advice. My sister found this very hard. I didn't care – it all seemed to go along in parallel to my real life. I wasn't full of resentment or hatred. I knew the name of the anaesthetic consultant involved in my case, although I had never met her. I wanted her to fully appreciate what she had done to me. After all, she had never even attempted to say sorry.

I did find it difficult that my sister had reservations about suing the hospital. She tells me she felt embarrassed and alone as a medical student and soon-to-be junior doctor. Her colleagues often chatted about how claims against the NHS were sapping the institution dry. They were invariably seen as ill-founded money grabs in a society obsessed with apportioning blame and making a quick buck. She also felt anxious that she herself might make a mistake and end up in court, and it would be her just desserts. Later she came to believe that the accident had changed her attitudes as a medic. She had learnt what it is to be an anguished relative, the essence of good and bad communication, and how the latter can foster ill-feeling and paranoia in the patient and their loved ones, and she had first-hand experience of the intricacies of a medical negligence claim. These had all helped her to become a better doctor, she felt, but they were all skills that she could never talk about to anyone but her closest friends. They were things she never discussed with work colleagues, and neither was she able to bring them to an interview table, since she felt that to do so would alienate her, leading to her being cast as emotionally vulnerable, arrogant or a troublemaker.

Rose admits she had a good reason to want to believe everything was OK: it was a possible way to persuade us not to go ahead with the legal case. She felt she had no choice but to keep the nature of my accident to herself. Her explanation was no help. All I could feel was that she was embarrassed by what had happened to me. She was embarrassed by me. Our relationship was under strain.

My sister believes that my accident changed her personality. Once a shy retiring thing, she could now have a flaming row with anyone and often did, especially with my aunties and uncles. She hated people asking her how I was: to her this was a false show of sympathy. She would give some kind of conventionally acceptable and polite response – 'Oh, she's doing well' – but felt like shouting: 'Why are you asking me? Ask her yourself. Antoinette is not dumb!'

My mother responded by avidly reading all the books she could find on head injury. She was aware of the mental health problems I might experience and this worried her; she well knew the stigma it might bring. She was convinced that intensive rehabilitation for the first year at least, and then vocational training of some sort, was the best chance I stood of recovering some normality. Yet this kind of prolonged rehabilitation was only available in the USA or privately in the UK, and we just could not afford the kind of money the institutions were asking for. One thing my mum was clear on was that I would not go into an assisted living facility just yet. She finally found a private place in Godalming, Surrey, called Unsted Park, and then worked to persuade the powers that be that my place should be funded as there was no equivalent in the NHS. It is only now that I come to write my story that I begin to appreciate the amount of work Mum put in to get me into the various rehabilitation facilities.

My mother insisted on reminding people, close friends and professionals, that I was not the well adult I appeared to be – I had suffered a significant brain injury. To her this was a pure statement of fact. To me it had no real meaning or impact. To the hearer (and even more so to my sister) it seemed my mother was being harsh and derogatory. People would tell her off, saying she shouldn't say such things in my hearing, yet it was probably she who understood the situation better than anyone.

To many friends and family I was a physically well woman in her mid-twenties. I was an adult. My family had to let go and I had to 'live my life', make my own mistakes – the problem was that my life had stopped that February day in 1995. I had no idea how to live my life. I displayed all the frustration and confusion of an angst-ridden teenager, at once wanting my family to leave me alone and to hold my hand, to guide me, to show they loved me. It was an impossible situation for them, and the idea of me learning from my mistakes was both cruel and fruitless in my parents' eyes. I had suffered enough, and anyway, as my mum explained, who was to say I would learn any lessons, let alone the right lessons, from my errors?

If my father was the dreamer and clown, my mother was very much the practical one. She had always been outspoken, taking on causes and fighting injustice, even if it made her unpopular with people because she highlighted their shortcomings and ignorance. But I have to say, although it is painful to admit it (only joking, Mum), she has rarely been wrong in her assessments. My illness and rehabilitation consumed my mother. She fought for me at every turn; she says she felt she was fighting a battle on her own, receiving

47

painful criticism at every step – from me, from my sister, from her husband, from friends, and sometimes from health professionals. But deep down she was confident she knew her daughter better than anyone, even better than her daughter knew herself by this stage.

By 1996 my mum had become ill, being diagnosed with sarcoidosis. This is an inflammatory condition, the cause of which is unknown; she is convinced that its ferocity and speed of onset were due to the stress she was under. The sarcoidosis affected her eyes, her spinal cord, her skin, her lungs. She was seriously ill, and we thought she might well die.

I finished at Northwick Park in August 1995, and my parents decided to take me to Lourdes in France for some more divine intervention. It seemed as if God hadn't quite finished the job and needed a little reminder that I was still in need of His attention. So we took a three-day excursion via Eurostar. I remember lots of people in wheelchairs, and drizzly rain. My sister asked me recently what I felt: I felt nothing. On our return my parents were secretly very worried as they were at a loss as to what would be the next step in my recuperation. I am convinced our desperate prayers worked, as within an hour of returning home I got a call from Dr Michael Oddy to say that my application to continue rehabilitation at Unsted Park had been accepted. Unsted Park is a private rehabilitation centre located in Godalming, and part of the well-known Priory group of health establishments popular with the rich and famous.

Chapter 5

More rehabilitation

I liked Unsted Park. It was a magnificent place, a beautiful stately home in the middle of the Surrey countryside, with private grounds and its own highland cattle and resident ghost. Patients whose rooms were in the old part of the house would tell me about knocks on their doors in the middle of the night by an invisible phantom. Apparently it is the ghost of the woman who lived in the house 60 years ago. She had been pushed off the third-floor balcony and had fallen three storeys before she smashed into the smoking room floor. She had been pushed by her husband – typical!

I had a structured day, starting in the morning with orientation when clients and therapists would all sit down together. We would state in turn who we were, what our goals were for the day and what was on the timetable. We would also discuss a recent news event. During the week I would have occupational therapy sessions in which I learnt to cook such staples as macaroni cheese. We did physical activities, such as swimming or walks around the grounds. There were individual speech and language therapy sessions – for me the aim was to improve my word-finding skills – and psychology sessions as well. All this mental and physical exertion were offset by mealtimes, when waiters in bow ties served us scrumptious three-course meals. Suddenly you felt you were in a five-star resort, not a rehabilitation facility. This was a definite plus for me.

Every Thursday Dr Oddy, who was based at the sister unit in Ticehurst, would come and give a lecture on the nature of brain injury. One day he drew a picture of the brain and I correctly named each lobe and region, even going on to say that the two halves of the brain were connected by the corpus callosum. I was so proud of myself, and I am sure he was impressed too. I loved these lectures. I took notes and it made me feel like I was practising for going back to medical school. In the evening I sat and chatted to the other clients, or watched television. I was the only girl there. I think there were just five of us at the time with head injuries, although there were others receiving private rehab for physical disabilities. The other clients were all older, mostly having had strokes. One client had suffered a serious car accident. He was very funny, always joking and making inappropriate advances to the female nursing staff. In reality these were all signs of the frontal lobe damage he had suffered, which meant he could be disinhibited and lewd in his conversation, but he didn't bother or scare me. I liked him a lot; he made me smile. It was clear he had had some high-powered job when he was well. He kept saying how he was waiting for his fiancée to come back so he could go home. I later found out that his fiancée had actually left him, unable to cope with the change in his personality and behaviour – the same behaviour I found so amusing.

However much I enjoyed Unsted Park once I had finally resigned myself to being there for the week, I hated Sunday evenings and would refuse to go back to the unit. It was rather like the abject distress you feel as a child the day before the new school year starts. I would cry, begging my parents not to take me back. 'Please, let me just stay at home,' I would implore them. My parents would try to coax me by joining me for my evening meal to try to calm me down. I also was playing along, and would plead again at the end of the meal: 'Right, can we go home now?' Sundays never got any easier throughout the eight months I was at Unsted Park, and returning after Christmas was trebly hard.

One important lesson I learned at Unsted Park was to avoid alcohol. Dr Oddy told us the decision was finally ours, allowing us to weigh up the pros and cons. Many of the brain-injured people I have met do drink for many of the same social reasons that most young people drink – to improve self-esteem and confidence, to keep up with peers and be socially acceptable – but added to this is drinking because of sheer boredom. We all know the consequences of too much alcohol: making us more disinhibited and more likely to attempt risky activities, slowing our responses. As my mum used to say to me, she didn't want me to pickle the neurons I had left.

I know I drank too much before the accident, so I am very pleased that I manage to avoid alcohol altogether now. I do miss it, and often used to sniff a glass of wine to get the taste of some of those tannins from the vapour. However, my taste buds are now more accustomed to the sweetness of Diet Coke. I have had to learn how to socialise without alcohol, which is possible although not easy. In the beginning, when my social skills were poor, if my monosyllabic answers didn't kill the conversation then saying I didn't want to drink because I'd had a head injury certainly put the nail in the coffin. But in spite of this, I really do believe that to drink alcohol is pure foolishness for someone who has suffered a brain injury. The only downside is that when I am bored I get my instant gratification by shopping instead, which is no good for the bank balance.

On leaving Unsted Park in the summer of 1996, I was on a high. I thought the world was my oyster. Having learnt the daily skills of life and believing I had mastered them, I thought that resuming a 'normal' life was going to be a piece of cake. In reality it was more as if my life had turned into a plate of crumbs and I was left to pick up the pieces. I naively thought I would magically resume my studies and everything would fall into place. I did not acknowledge that I was OK only when I took things at my own speed, but struggled badly if someone else was setting the pace.

There was no part of me that consciously accepted or believed my brain had changed, that it was not able to do now what it had done so effortlessly before. Even during my stints in rehab there seemed to be part of me that played along with all the therapists because it was what was expected of me while another part was biding its time to get back to my old life. One did not impact on the other. Maybe others would call this lack of insight. My dad always promised me that my life would be better than it had been, and I was holding on to his promise. With hindsight, now, I don't really blame my dad, but it was lack of knowledge about brain injury and wishful thinking on his part that fuelled his early 'everything will be alright in the end' attitude. My elation was short-lived. My mother was seriously ill with sarcoidosis, and come the August of that year I felt so desperate that I took a drug overdose.

I returned home from Unsted Park, waiting to resume my medical training, which the new dean of the college said I could attempt with the next academic intake in 1998. But because the course had changed so much, and because of my long leave of absence, he said I could only resume my training if I started again from the first year. I was not impressed. I had done all this before! My mother had known for a while that medicine would be a hard slog and was really not sure if I could manage it. The dean's decision was actually a welcome relief to her. But she kept her worries to herself. She had been told by all around, especially my dad and my sister, to leave me alone, on the one hand accused of mothering me and holding me back and on the other portrayed as a typical overbearing Asian mother who must be pushing her daughter into medicine.

In the summer of 1997 my sister got married. It was a happy time and my mood was good. I had worked through the suicidal thoughts of the previous summer, and though Mum was still ill she had come through the doctor's initial fears. All summer was abuzz with wedding plans, and relatives and friends were coming from the United States and Canada. I was bridesmaid, and felt useful. Dad had insisted that I start driving again (I had swapped my manual for an automatic, which was a lot easier to drive), so I helped ferry my relatives around. I had one car accident that shook me up, but otherwise life was quite good. To cap it all, one of my sister's friends who was at the wedding and had visited me a few times in hospital decided he liked me enough to want to start going out with me. I was thrilled. My life seemed to have turned a corner.

I decided to go travelling just like I had done in my gap year before starting at St Mary's. I would travel for six months, visiting my aunts and uncles in the States and Canada. Though some made it to the wedding, many had not seen me since my accident and my time in intensive care. I wanted to remove that image from their minds, and show them that not only had I recovered but I was a new and improved Antoinette.

I used often to ask my parents and my sister what I was like before the accident. They would tell me how they were a bit anxious about my partying and drinking; it was not very Sri Lankan and not very Christian. They did not know what to do, and in a funny way they believed the accident had put the brakes on my behaviour. This was the good that would come out of the bad. I couldn't believe I had become so wayward, and for many years I felt my accident had come as a punishment for all my worldly excesses. God had given me a second chance, and I promised myself and Him that I was going to be a different kind of person.

Generally I felt the trip was a resounding success. Some family friends refused to have me visit them as they thought I might behave oddly or have a fit and scare their children. This upset my family enormously, but fortunately it was a rare response. I helped for a couple of hours a week in a laboratory in the Texas hospital where my uncle was a surgeon. I also watched him do a few operations. The holiday was not a sightseeing tour. Many of my relatives were out at work in the daytime and this gave me ample time to rest and discover a substitute for *Neighbours* in the form of *Sunset Beach*, a glamorous Californian soap opera with outrageously improbable storylines featuring pretty maidens in comas and dastardly evil twins (it had a cult following in the UK, I later discovered). I don't know what my relatives thought of me – maybe that I was quiet, I don't know. I have a feeling my mother had tipped them off.

Once I babysat my cousin Maureen's two children, JR and Mitchell; they were five and three at the time. I bathed them, got them dressed in their night clothes and settled them into bed. I was exhausted but very pleased with myself and went off to bed myself for a well-deserved sleep. My cousin returned to find me sound asleep and the children happily awake – and thankfully OK. Maureen was kind enough to see the funny side.

I enjoyed meeting my cousins, but it was hard to know that those younger than me were doing so well at university. In my eyes the benchmark to my recovery was returning to medicine and qualifying as a doctor, and since I had not achieved that yet, meeting my younger cousins was a painful experience.

Towards the end of the holiday I had a big fight with my uncle Wije – with hindsight, maybe it was the first sign that the mask of 'wellness' I had worn so diligently was actually starting to slip. I had got into a complete panic about not having enough luggage space. I needed a new bag, and I needed it now. The fact that my uncle had just stepped through the door from a ten-hour day at work and a two-hour commute did not concern me. He couldn't understand why I was getting into such a state. I was frantic; I wanted to be back home. My uncle was shaken by what had happened. He had never seen me behave like this before – it scared him. After I returned home he decided to do some reading on head injury and got himself a copy of a book called *Over My Head* by Claudia Osborn, a medic who had suffered a traumatic brain injury after being thrown off her bike in a collision with a car.

I returned to England on Boxing Day 1997, and plummeted into a deep depression. I felt physically drained, as if I was running on empty. Maybe I had called on reserves of sociability I hadn't known I needed in order to make my holiday the resounding success I so desperately wanted it to be. Maybe it was a reaction to returning to an empty house and realising that my life could not be a continuous holiday. Noxious fumes of deep hopelessness filled the empty vacuum, and my mind toyed with ways to uncork this pressurised vessel. I finally admitted to my mother that I had thoughts of harming myself, of cutting my wrists. It was a great disappointment to her. The holiday had seemed like such a big step forward, a sign that I was well on the road to recovery, but my admission raised all the fears of the previous summer, and my sessions with the psychologist duly increased.

I had nearly ten months to fill before university started. Mum had secured support for me from a neuropsychologist based at Garston Manor, an outpatient facility for brain-injured people near my home. I was probably one of their last clients as I am led to believe it became a plush wedding venue later that year. I decided to work on an A level in human biology at the local college. I had also put myself down to do psychology and sociology, but unfortunately my head injury had failed to make these subjects any more interesting so I gave them up after a semester. I managed to get a B in my A level that year. I took on voluntary roles for a couple of hours a week – one day at a nursing home and one day at a local hospital, being a befriender to residents and patients. I filled out menu cards and at the nursing home made teas and coffees, coordinated activities and chatted to the residents.

I still found social interactions with my peers very difficult. I didn't particularly want to go out, especially as I was now depressed, and my voluntary work was undertaken more under duress than because I was keen to occupy myself – my psychologist had advised me I should do it. I had episodes of rage during this time. I had regular headaches, and bad cramps if I overdid it. I think I did get some enjoyment from the work, but I rarely spoke to my family about what I did all day, just coming home tired and keen to head straight to bed. They must have liked me there, though, because I got some lovely leaving gifts, including an ornamental china plate with kittens painted on it that takes pride of place on my dressing table, as well as some sincere best wishes for the restart of my medical degree.

On the days when I was not doing voluntary work, it had been arranged for a psychology student to come and visit me at home to help me organise my day. I told her to go away; I didn't need her help. My life was quite lonely. I had no contact with my old medical school mates and had made no new friends. My boyfriend did try to get me out of the house, and this really helped my family. My sister told me things would get better when I was back at college and meeting people of my own age again.

Chapter 6

What is brain injury?

There are a number of books about brain injury, and I have given the names of a few at the end of this book, but if you are anything like me there are two reasons why you might not read up about head injury: (1) it has nothing to do with you, or so you tell yourself; (2) the books are too long and boring. So here is my potted 'idiot's guide' to head injury.

There are lots of different types of brain injury. You can be born with it, usually because of being starved of oxygen in the womb, or you can acquire it. Acquired brain injury often results from a trauma such as a car accident or an assault. Many of my friends acquired their brain injury this way, as either drivers, passengers, cyclists, pedestrians or bystanders, all being in the wrong place at the wrong time. Head injuries are a big social problem as the adults most likely to be affected are those in the prime of life, often in their twenties, and they are most often men, who are likely to be more risk-taking in their behaviour.

Most head injuries happen in children but they generally seem to have the ability to recover better than adults. Worryingly, alcohol seems to have some part to play in how the majority of adult brain injuries are acquired: for example, the drunk driver who mows down a pedestrian, or the inebriated student who falls off a fourth-storey window ledge while standing outside for a quick smoke.

My kind of brain injury, caused by a lack of oxygen to the brain due to a cardiac arrest, is also a type of acquired brain injury, as are certain medical illnesses such as a stroke, bleed or tumour. Many people who have direct traumatic brain injury have what is known as 'closed' injury – in other words, the skull is not broken yet the brain has been given a good shaking about and may even have bruised itself on the hard, jagged skull interior. Unfortunately it is the frontal lobes (which are the seat of our personality) and our temporal lobes (which are involved with memory) that seem to suffer the most, even with what could be regarded as a mild trauma.

For some reason it seems that, whatever the cause of the brain injury, we all suffer profound tiredness, headaches, mood changes and sometimes muscle cramps, especially in the early weeks and months, although these symptoms can persist for years. If the damage is due to a direct blow to the head or a blood clot then you may have weakness down one side, problems with the way you speak or impairment of your vision, depending on which bit of the brain has been injured, because different parts of the brain coordinate different things. In addition, damaged nerves can fire abnormally, placing you at risk of epileptic fits.

In my case I didn't have a direct blow, and no one bit of my brain was specifically injured. As a result, I don't have any problems with my walking or talking as such. But because my brain was 'generally' starved of oxygen, those areas of my brain that are most sensitive – such as the hippocampus, which deals with memory and learning along with the temporal lobes, and the basal ganglia, which deal with movement – seem to have been damaged (possibly the reason why I had all those involuntary movements in intensive care). My memory has improved a little over the years but it is unlikely to get much better from now on. I also know that whereas once I grasped ideas and knowledge quickly, I now struggle to learn anything new. I am aware that my memory may also start to get worse more quickly with age than the memories of those who have not had an injury.

The funny thing is that even a minor head injury can cause severe memory problems – the brain is a very complex organ. I have problems with memory, especially in terms of spoken language, so I am no good at remembering telephone conversations. Please don't ask me why I decided to take a job in the John Lewis call centre after leaving Westminster Council! Needless to say, it was short-lived; in fact, I lasted just a few hours before my boss took me off the phones as the customers were getting so irate.

Also I can no longer do that one thing women pride themselves in, namely multitasking. If I get information coming at me from different sources, my brain shuts down. This can either make me react with anger or, more often, turn me into a nervous, blithering lump of jelly. My sister says I look like a startled rabbit, moving one way then the other, my heart racing, my actions frantic but fruitless. At other times I just freeze and switch off – I think this is what other people with head injury describe as flooding.

The ability to multitask is an example of the higher executive functions a brain carries out. My family say I display a number of problems in this area. It is something that has not improved with time for me. My family and I are just more aware now of how to keep me out of situations where I need to multitask, and then I manage OK.

The cerebral cortex also seems to affect our social behaviour. I know that after the accident I had terrible problems with feelings of anger, and could fly off the handle very quickly. In the early years I didn't know how to modulate my voice, so it seemed as though I was shouting out answers to innocuous questions like 'How are you?' I know my impulsivity is a form of disinhibition caused by changes in my frontal lobes. I have friends who just can't stop talking, saying every idea that comes into their heads. In some ways it could be liberating not to be bound by these social niceties that have ensnared us since toddlerhood. The problem is that we still have to make it in the real world where people can see us as odd, or worse.

It seems that, whatever the cause of your brain injury, these executive functions are always affected to a greater or lesser degree and for a variable length of time. Executive functions seem to be the latest in our evolutionary development, marking us out as complex social beings, but seem to be the most vulnerable to attack. My sister says it may be because we in the developed world aspire to intellectual jobs, getting higher qualifications and working in managerial roles, so the effects of a brain injury on our ability to work tend to be that much more apparent and devastating than if we were all unskilled labourers.

The executive functions I am describing include the ability to make plans, to see those plans through, to monitor our activities, to see the bigger picture, to think laterally about how to achieve a certain goal, and to do more than one thing at a time. All this is difficult for me, and made worse by my inability to concentrate, especially if any element of stress or tiredness is added. I operate extremely impulsively, especially when I am not depressed and am generally happy with life! When I am depressed I do nothing except feel anxious. I can feel on a high and make sudden decisions without thinking through the risks and benefits. I can suddenly decide I like reading, or want to make jewellery, and then go on to spend quite a lot of money on books or beads, only for my interest to wane within a few weeks. This again is a change from who I was before the accident, as I had always been very methodical by nature.

Probably one of the reasons why I talk about who I was before the accident is because who I am now is not so very different from how many people without brain injury are – I never got a university degree, I am hopeless with money and I live a chaotic, impulsive, sometimes volatile life. The only problem is that this is not who I was: I was a different type of person. My family still remember the old me, and hence it has taken them and me a long time to get to know the new

Antoinette. To be honest, I don't remember what I was like before the accident – I remember incidents and events, but not how I thought. It's like remembering your childhood. You are transported to a different time but you look and feel the same as you do today. I am 30 years old and five feet two inches, in a playground with my ten-year-old friends. I know I was different because of what others tell me, but I cannot even contemplate being any person other than who I am today or even who I am in this moment. Yet I am often dogged by an uneasy sense that, no, things are not quite right – but I can't quite put my finger on what has changed.

When I say I have memory problems, many people say, 'Yes, so do I. My memory is rubbish – I always have to make lists.' The problem with my memory is that I forget to even make the list, and if I do make a list I usually forget to look at it. In an odd way I am more likely to remember the mundane parts of my life, or a feeling or emotion, than something important like a hospital appointment. My sister gets so annoyed with me when she asks me to do something and I invariably say, 'Wait, I need to write this down.' I have a pen in my bag but not my writing pad. 'Can I get an envelope out of your recycling bin?' I of course then lose the envelope on which I have written my note. She now texts me anything really important on the day I need to do it. She then calls or texts me to check that I have done it. I asked once, in rather a hurt tone, if she trusted me. She answered, matter-of-factly, 'No.'

I know comments like, 'Oh, I have a bad memory too,' are well-meaning, trying to show some degree of understanding and empathy, but in reality they often undermine the very experience that I and others like me are having. This is not a bit of dippy forgetfulness, difficulty with names and birthdays. The reality is that my head injury has taken away my career, my friends, my personality; it has taken away the old me. That is not to say that I feel angry about these

61

comments. They upset me for a day, but then the great thing about a bad memory is that I forget what was said, even if not the feeling, in record time – there has to be some silver lining to my dark cloud!

I still struggle sometimes to believe that there is anything wrong with me as I look so well physically, so it doesn't surprise me that others can't really understand what I am experiencing. I am convinced that no one can properly understand what we who have suffered brain injury experience until – heaven forbid – they experience such an injury themselves.

I think the other hidden and little-talked-about effect of brain injury is that it can leave us as vulnerable adults, all the more so if we are unaware of our deficiencies. Sometimes the only people who see our vulnerability are family members. This puts a particular strain on relationships, as we, the brain-injured, try to exert our independence while our families work even harder to protect us from what they see as a cruel world, and maybe even from ourselves. I know my family have found it difficult to know when to pull back, knowing not only that this will allow me to make mistakes but that they may only hear about a mistake when the problem is out of control.

I am fortunate in that I do now have some insight into my problems, insight that has grown over the years and with the many less-than-happy situations I have found myself in. I am aware that my brain injury has left me with a childlike ability to trust anyone who is kind to me, even if I know very little about them. I tend to see in black and white; I often don't see grey, and I usually don't recognise ulterior motives or inconsistent behaviour. This also means that when new people come into my life I often turn to them in preference to my family, as part of my overwhelming desire to be normal, adult and independent. These are always times of great stress for my family, as they watch from the sidelines, desperately hoping I don't get hurt, exploited or ridiculed.

Chapter 7

Back to medicine

The week before starting university, I excitedly flicked through my freshers' packs and all the other paraphernalia that had arrived through the letterbox. It was October 1998. I think I was like a bubble on the verge of bursting, I was so excited. I remembered my first freshers' week well and was just as keen and eager this second time around. I bought a freshers' week bumper entrance card to get me into all the ice-breaking social events and bops that had been arranged. I was certainly not going to miss out on any of the fun.

The pass proved to be a waste of money. The harsh reality was that I struggled to go to even one event owing to sheer exhaustion from the day itself. This upset me. I had always imagined I could pick up where I had left off, and that everything would be rosy! But I had been kidding myself, and with my fatigue levels greatly increased, I was incapable of enduring even short activities. I would be so physically and mentally exhausted after a day of lectures or practicals that it was as much as I could do to get myself back to halls and to my bed. My legs ached, going into painful spasms; my head pounded, and I had no energy or even the wherewithal to get myself something to eat. My family visited most evenings to check how I was doing. They would try to make sure I had eaten, and would settle me into bed before making the twenty-mile journey home. Getting tucked into bed by my parents was not the student life I had remembered. Why was I struggling so much?

Since my first time around as a medical student, St Mary's, along with Charing Cross Hospital Medical School, had been absorbed into Imperial College, and the lectures were held across all three sites. I often got confused as to where I should be, and would end up at the wrong place or just go back to my halls, exhausted. My tutors were concerned about why I was not interacting at all in tutorials. The truth was that I couldn't keep up. The discussion, the flow of ideas, was like a tidal wave. When I did come up with something to say, it took me a little while to formulate the words in my head and meanwhile the topic had moved on. My brain could not handle more than a few minutes of information before switching off, my head swirling in the deluge of those tidal waters. I would carefully tape all my lectures so that I could listen to them in the evenings, but I rarely played them again.

Why wasn't I able to do the things I had once found so routine and easy? When it came to my studies, my memory was not the sponge I had once relied on. It had become a colander, with information leaking out faster than I could put it in. As I struggled to manage my day and my exhausted evening, in which I would usually go to bed early with fatigue, cramps and a migraine, I started to decline into depression. I had been on antidepressants since a year after my accident. My GP at the time said that it was silly for me be on them and that I would become dependent if I didn't start to come off them soon. Strangely, many brain-injured people find that they need antidepressants throughout their whole life.

I physically, emotionally and psychologically limped through that first year. Most nights I would call my family in distress, and call again in the early hours of the morning in a blind panic as to how I would face another day. Sometimes I was calling four or five times during the night. I had been taught relaxation techniques, but none would work now. Once I was near hysterical as I didn't seem to be able to adjust my hi-tech Posturepaedic chair, and my boyfriend travelled across London in the early hours of the morning to try to sort things out for me. With hindsight I know that sometime during that year my motivation changed, and I endured the rest of the year not because I was dying to be a medic any more but because I wanted to prove the neurologists and neuropsychologists wrong. But they were right! I would struggle to study anything, even a basic degree course.

My psychologist from Garston Manor had arranged ongoing psychology support for me, so while my classmates spent Wednesday afternoons on the river or sports field, I went to Charing Cross to talk about how the week had gone and what I could do to tackle the problems I had experienced. My psychologist also spoke to my tutor so that she was up to speed with my progress.

Once my sister decided to join me. It was nice to have her company. We came out of Barons Court tube and walked through the cemetery. I told my sister how I found Hammersmith cemetery peaceful, and she agreed – it felt as though we were miles from the busy-ness of the flyover, possibly the worst bit of highway in London. When she came with me it was springtime, and the huge cherry tree at the entrance to the cemetery was heavy with blossom. The cemetery was full of old headstones, huge carved angels praying over their deceased charges, giving the place an other-worldly quality.

As we climbed the steps to Charing Cross hospital I mentioned in passing to my sister that my psychologist was in the same clinic as those awaiting gender reassignment – I thought she had better know. I had been attending the clinic for months; nothing had the power to shock me, and it had never occurred to me to let anyone know, even as a little bit of an interesting aside, who my Wednesday afternoon companions were. My sister was impressed and intrigued. She waited in the waiting room while I went in for my session. Seeing the clinic through her eyes did make me smile at the irony – the sight of two slightly scruffy, short, un-made-up Asian girls in a room full of predominantly six-foot burly individuals dressed in very short miniskirts, or else looking like surly librarians from the 1970s with satin blouses, pearls and oversized spectacles. Most had beautifully manicured fingernails on the ends of spade-like hands, and size twelve patent stilettos. My sister looked at her clothes with a slight degree of concern as we were leaving. She has never been one to be overly concerned with her appearance, and shopping brings her out in hives.

'Do you think people might think we are here to become men?' she asked, with some concern.

'I don't know,' I replied flatly. 'They probably don't care'.

In spite of my best efforts and unstinting support from everyone around me, I failed all my first-year exams, even though they gave me permission to take each exam separately from everyone else so I would not feel distracted. I was given extra time and an amanuensis (or scribe) in case I should find it difficult to write, as I used to get bad muscle cramps in my hands if I wrote for too long. It was a bitter blow. I was scheduled to sit the retakes in August. I slaved tirelessly throughout my whole summer break, borrowing a close friend's notes and spending hours, usually from 7.30 am until about 10 pm, reading and doing practice multiple-choice quizzes at the end of the revision of each topic. I loved quizzes, but not this type! My sister helped by going through multiple-choice questions with me on the computer, but even she was anxious at how little information I was retaining.

On retaking my medicine exams, which consisted of two three-hour multiple-choice papers plus one essay paper and a problem-based learning paper on colon cancer (I passed that one at least), I was short-listed for a pass/fail viva (oral examination with the head of faculty) on the other three papers. Seeing my number on the pass/fail viva list broke me. I caved in under the enormity of what I had endured over the year and simply couldn't face any more. I had had enough. I knew I wouldn't be going back to Imperial College come

October. My identity as a hard-working, fun-loving medical student had been stripped bear – an identity I had cherished for so long. I know part of my fighting spirit left me that summer.

During the course of a weekend in August 1999, I enrolled for a radiotherapy degree at City University. I have to say that one thing I have rarely struggled with is making myself look good on paper, and to a lesser degree making myself look good at interview. They accepted me straight away. With hindsight, I know that my impulsive style of decision-making is perhaps not the best possible way of deciding on these crucial choices!

I commenced my radiotherapy degree. The lectures were good; I had covered most of the material many times before and, for once, I felt one step ahead of my peers. In the last four weeks of that first semester, the students had to do the clinical component. I was sent to St Bartholomew's Hospital near the Barbican in London. I recall setting off for my eight o'clock start in the radiotherapy wing in the basement of the hospital (most radiography and radiotherapy equipment is stored in the basement, surrounded by concrete and earth, to guard against the risk of a radiation leak). I struggled through the first day, having to think and calculate radiation doses on my feet and running from one radiation suite to another. Come five o'clock, to say that I was 'pooped' is putting it mildly. I returned to my hall of residence exhausted. However, sleep eluded me; my legs were in painful spasm and my head pounded. The next morning, dead on my feet, I went and spoke to my tutor and excused myself from the course. I don't think he was too upset or surprised. He had really thought I was having a nervous breakdown. For my part, I knew my accident had been the result of someone's mistake, and I did not want to be the cause of another mistake at the expense of an individual in my care.

I slumped into a depression. With my depressions I get severely anxious, waking at four or five each morning only to suffer a few hours more of nervous anxiety. Oddly, I don't become tearful or introspective; I rarely seem to cry about anything. I have to keep checking if I have locked doors and windows, going back four, maybe five times. I might lie around all day but I wouldn't be sleeping. My appearance, which has always been important to me, would be of no consequence. My weight would go up along with the dose of my antidepressants.

After much cajoling from the family I enrolled on a nutrition and pharmacology degree at Luton University. It was one of the few modular courses on offer in the UK – modular meaning that I would not have to go through the stress of exams, which my brain just could not handle any more. Luton was definitely not my first choice, and I struggled with the fact I had once received offers from the likes of St Andrews. Luton was certainly a far cry from the world-famous Imperial College, University of London. The snobby side of me had helped me rise above the bullying I received as a child; now it was my undoing, as I was in danger of setting my sights too high and overestimating my abilities. I was accepted on the course, which was due to start in the following September.

I spent my time off volunteering in a home for the elderly, after which I holidayed in the United States, staying with family friends in New York. I have to say a special thank you to the O'Donnells: I used to love my stays with them. They always treated me as nothing less than an equal. They took me to theatres and art galleries, they talked to me about their favourite reads and treated me to dinner in their golf club. This was not done especially for me – I just slotted into their busy vibrant schedules. I walked daily through Central Park when I was in Manhattan, and once saw Harrison Ford walking to or from a game of tennis. New York is just beautiful at any time of year. Everyone talks fast and is so incredibly busy, but as a visitor you are not supposed to keep up. No one expects you to – I liked that. I returned to England in plenty of time to have a last chance at getting a qualification.

During this time the preparations for the court case continued. I had to see psychologists and neuropsychologists, for my side and then for the other side of the legal case. I read and reread the reports with morbid interest. My sister hated me to read these reports as she was convinced they were making me negative and pulling me down. But I think it was my sister who was more affected by them than I could ever be at that time. Reading them always put her in a very bad mood for days, so often she just ignored them. The tests and the results didn't mean anything to me, but the summary at the start of the reports that stated who I was and what had happened to me was always intriguing. I felt bound to, yet at the same time strangely detached from, the person they were speaking about. The reports always came back saying the same thing: that my chances of getting back into medicine were zero, and the most I would achieve would be a few hours of voluntary or unskilled paid work each week.

Chapter 8

Darkness my new friend

I had been on antidepressants since my accident. I have never been one to talk about my feelings. I had developed quite an independent streak as a child and had always managed to deal with the ups and downs of life that I had endured until my early adulthood. Pity parties were simply not my thing. Suddenly, I was experiencing flares of depression each February at the time of the anniversary of my accident. I also seemed to get generally down through the winter months. As my academic dreams, and then my vocational dreams, edged away from me, I slipped further into depression. I was having bouts of depression at least three or four times a year, possibly more. My most serious bouts occurred in the summer of 1996, in early 1998 after my grand tour of the States, and in 2005, when I finally had to acknowledge the extent of my disabilities.

In 1996 my mother had been diagnosed with sarcoidosis. This affected her skin, eyes, lungs and nervous system. She was seriously ill, needing treatment at the Royal Brompton Hospital. We had had what we thought might be our last holiday as a family that year. I found I resented my mother for being ill. I wanted to be independent and to be away from home, but also deep down I knew I desperately needed my family around. I felt my family had cheated me, that after all I had been through they had let me live only to leave me alone in the world. Sometimes in my anger I would accuse them of not caring about me. This was my harshest insult. I believed it, but I also knew it would hurt them deeply. Sometimes my words were like the vicious swipes and bites of a cornered and wounded animal.

My sister decided to get engaged in early 1996. She and John had been dating for over fifteen months. I had met John before my accident, but could not remember him from then and didn't particularly like him. He seemed to appear from nowhere, like a cuckoo in my nest (he is actually the best brother-in-law I could wish for). In August 1996 my sister was due to move out of the house to work as a junior doctor in Stevenage (John was going there too). The day before she started her new job I took my first overdose (my second was during the time after leaving my radiology course, and was probably more a cry for help than anything else).

My life was changing quicker than I could handle. My mother, who was still recovering and had only been discharged from hospital a few days earlier, did her best not to have me admitted to a psychiatric unit. My GP and the psychiatrist agreed that such a move would leave me labelled for life and would affect my still-expectant medical career. My mother, above anyone else, knows that although society is changing, the change is far from complete and mental illness is still one of society's greatest taboos. My mother's diabetes had worsened to become a significant health concern as a result of the steroid medication she was taking for her sarcoidosis. I chose to overdose on my mother's newly prescribed antidiabetic medication.

I gave the NHS a merry runaround that night. I had been taken to A&E in the family car, clutching a two-litre bottle of cherry Coke given to me by John to try to stave off the hypoglycaemic effects of the overdose. The consultant psychiatrist came down to the car park and tried coax me out of the car, promising I would not have to go to a psychiatric ward. I refused, but did agree to drink my Coke; I managed to drink the whole two-litre bottle. At four in the morning, now back at home and asleep next to my mother, I became severely unwell with hypoglycaemia – sweating, shaky and light-headed. My mother plied me with juice and somehow I made it through the day without slipping into a coma. I desperately wanted to die. This was no cry for help, but there must have been a part of me that would not let it happen. As my mum said, it would have been a sad thing if all I had managed to do was damage my brain even further.

The strain of the previous year, her own ill health and now the overdose frightened my mum, and she decided to get herself some counselling. The counsellor was clear in his assessment. By using my mother's tablets to overdose, I was giving out a clear message that I was trying to punish her. My mother was suddenly aware of the dangerous situation we as a family were facing, and this assessment made it even more evident to her that we needed outside help, that we couldn't just manage this situation on our own.

I know I related particularly badly to my mother. I also know this is a problem for daughters the world over, regardless of whether or not they have had a brain injury. But I can now see how my mother takes the brunt of my anger and frustration, and I do not think my response and relationship are unique. Moving back to a family home, having once been an independent adult, to be looked after by your parents creates problems and tensions not unique to those who have been brain-injured. Like all mums, she would try to provide practical solutions to the problems I faced, and this annoyed me. But my mother is also a psychiatrist. Her work was with offenders, drug addicts, alcoholics. She knew that how people perceived their environment could affect their behaviour, and that some destructive behaviours could become habits that were difficult to break. She was acutely aware of the implications of my words and feelings, implications I had no idea about. All I knew was that my relationship with her had an added element of difficulty, as I could not even open my mouth without her getting worried. Mum and I are each other's companions now, and she remains my only true confidante, but I can still resent the fact that she needs me as much as I need her. I see her walk slowly; she looks frail, and I feel angry with her for holding me up and interrupting my plans. At other times, when my anger has subsided, I feel desperately scared. I fear the very real possibility that I might lose her some day.

Over the next few years I had to adjust to the knowledge that I would never now become a doctor. Since the accident I have had fits of rage or fury. I don't know what precipitates them. I seem to have developed a very short fuse. This is one of the hardest changes that my family have had to deal with. As a child, though I was boisterous and loud, I was always known as the peacemaker. I hated shouting and upset. At the slightest sign of it I would silently cry, and rather like Tiny Tim in *A Christmas Carol*, with my sad countenance I would make everyone feel guilty enough to stop their silly quarrelling. Sometimes it was headaches and generally feeling worn out and unable to express myself adequately that made me shout. I wanted to be left alone, but desperately feared being abandoned. When I had my attacks of fury I would speak so fast that my words would just run into themselves. I didn't fully understand what I was saying or what I meant, so no one else could either.

I would be lying if I said that I wasn't angry with God. I was angry because I didn't deserve the health problems I had; I was angry because I had trusted that He had healed me, and yet I was not living the life I thought He wanted for me. I had not gone back to medicine, as people had promised me. I was not the new and improved version of my old self I had hoped to be. I was angry because church made no sense. The Bible made no sense; however hard I read it, I forgot it so fast. I was angry because I kept feeling so darn angry, and I just didn't know why.

My mother was aware that this was due to frontal lobe damage and a loss of emotional control. This knowledge was cold comfort, as it was with my mum that I often lost my rag.

My sister reacted less well. My parents couldn't believe their luck when as teenagers we seemed to get away with none of the tantrums and fights over clothing common in households of sisters. Instead, they were blessed with these rites of passage from their twenty-something daughters. Often after we had been out for an evening there would be a fight. My sister always felt she had to be watching over me, making sure I was OK and that I was interacting well, filling in any gaps in the conversation someone might have picked up with me, making sure that she could cover up if any tricky questions made me stumble and stall. By the end of the evening we would both be exhausted.

I never realised my sister was on this emotional roller coaster, constantly watching my reactions. I looked on oblivious, sometimes just lost in the noise and clatter of my surroundings. I would invariably be wearing my standard bemused frown. My sister took this to mean that I was angry with something she had done or said, or had failed to say or do. It is amazing how powerful non-verbal communication is. Not only had I lost the ability to pick up on others' non-verbal communication but I was communicating things that I didn't even realise I was feeling to those around me, without having any clue that I was doing so. The strain of these evenings was too much for either of us, and by the end we were both emotionally frazzled in our own ways. We would drive home silently, my mind a blank, hers ruminating on the evening's events and what they meant.

'What's wrong with you now?' she would ask accusingly as we went into the house. 'Your face looked like a thunder cloud the whole evening.'

My mum's smiles and hopes that we had had a pleasant day out would vanish as she let us in and could instantly sense that there would be an evening of door-slamming.

'What? Just go away. Nothing's wrong,' I would retort, my arms folded and my whole posture closed off.

'Well, it doesn't look like nothing.' She would be starting to get angry. 'We fall over backwards trying to help you, and you never say thank you – you never do anything.'

'Oh, just shut up. I suppose it would have been far better for you all if I had just died. Then you could carry on with you lives.'

'Yes, maybe we could, but we can't – we're trapped too.'

'Huh. Look at you. "Oh I am a doctor. I know everything. I am so clever",' I would say mockingly, swinging my shoulders from side to side, my chest puffed out. 'Well, I've never met anyone so heartless as you. I wish you knew what it was like to be me.' I couldn't even remember how this fight had started.

'Stop being so self-pitying. You're not a child – you need to get a grip.'

'Just shut up. I hate you! I hate you!'

Then I would run up the stairs to my room. My head would be pounding, my thoughts all jumbled. It felt similar to being on the point of passing out, but the feeling would last for what seemed like an age, made all the worse by the pounding headache I would invariably develop.

'Rose, leave her alone,' my mum would implore, grabbing her arm. 'Leave her alone.'

I could hear them go back downstairs. 'I need you to be friends, not fighting like this. Rose, she needs you. You have so much, and she has nothing'

'She hates me – you heard her. I know her life is ruined but I didn't do it to her. I can't help how things are'

'She knows that and she doesn't hate you.'

I could hear Rose sobbing downstairs. I knew Mum was crying too. In the darkness of the room I could feel the tears rolling down my face, into my ears and down the side of my neck, to be soaked up by my pillow. Finally sleep and a new day would come.

My family almost dreaded the times when my various periods of rehabilitation finished and I was home again. They knew that once I was at home I would quickly slip into an unmotivated state. My sister would ask me to read, but I had a pat answer for anything that smacked of instruction: 'No, I'm too tired.' I was very aware of my loneliness, but I could in no way think of what it was I needed to do to help my situation. I saw things at one point in time only. I saw the happy loving family; I saw people chatting and laughing, and I resented them. Why did my life have to be so much harder than theirs?

My family tried to explain that these things take time, so for example to enjoy chatting maybe I needed to read a book or see a film to act as a focus for a conversation. This irritated me. Coming from my family it sounded like a lecture, and taken as such it was resisted with all my being: 'Books give me a headache and I forget the story. Films are the same.' Were they stupid or something? Had they forgotten I had had a brain injury? Once my sister bought me a Brain Training computer game, convinced that using quizzes to try to improve my memory would be good. She remembers my look of disappointment as I gave back her gift and said, as though revealing some deep part of me, 'Rose, I can't do quizzes. My memory is no good.'

My family worried about the weight I was putting on as a result of my physical inactivity. After all, my heart had taken a severe battering, and the extra weight made my joints ache. In spite of my medical background, I had lost the ability to rationalise my symptoms, to know what I needed to do to keep myself healthy. All aches and pains scared me. I was and still am desperately frightened of being ill, of being stabbed with needles and of history repeating itself.

Sometimes it felt that a swift death would be a better result. I would go to visit my GP almost weekly with some complaint. There was little he could do (remember, I can't take paracetamol or ibuprofen). He would listen and gently nod, and then I would go home.

My family tried to encourage me to walk. In the early years this brought on spasms, but they knew I had managed when the physiotherapists were there to make me. Yet again, this advice coming from my family was seen by me as just another attempt to find fault. It made me believe they didn't love me or even like me. In fact, this was probably more a reflection of how I felt about myself. Well, I didn't care what they thought of me, and I definitely would not be exercising!

Mum was aware that for my family to try to advise me was just not working. Our relationships were showing the strain, and might well disintegrate completely. She would go to my GP saying, 'We need help. We can't be her therapists.' My mother wanted me to see a clinical psychologist at least, even if I was not in full rehab. She felt it would get me out of the house and allow me to explore my feelings, so that I didn't develop any 'bad habits', as she put it. I had already expressed feelings of wanting to cut my wrists after returning from my holiday in America, and my mother was aware that there was a good chance I might develop drink or drug habits as an abnormal way of coping with my situation. These ideas had to be nipped in the bud before they were acted on.

I have seen clinical psychologists almost without a break since my accident, mostly funded privately, though sometimes we did get them on the NHS. They would make regular contact with my family to see how I was doing at home. Often I would talk to my mum about how I felt, only to forget to bring it up come my therapy session. My family were also aware that I would not be honest about my deficits, not because I was trying to deceive but because I didn't recognise them as such, and because I had developed every excuse under the sun to explain away any erratic behaviour on my part. A good line of communication between my family and my therapist was essential for all of us, or else the therapy would be a waste of time.

My therapist would bring up with me any concerns my family had raised with her, so we could discuss them in the sessions. I was given assignments, like going for a walk or watching a film, and I had either to do them or explain why I hadn't in the next session. It was generally easier for me just to do them. Every time I had to change therapists, either because I had moved to college or because they had a change in personal circumstances, it was a cause of great anxiety for my family. My family depended on my therapists to give me sensible advice and to guide me, since it was clear I would not take advice from the family. I have to admit that, although I know that I went to them, I remember little of what we discussed. I am sure some of my therapists got fed up with the fact that, though I seemed eager to take on board all their good advice, I never managed to implement more than a couple of strategies. I seemed to have lost my ability to persist with a task. However, with hindsight I think my mum was right: the therapy session did allow me an opportunity to learn how to express my feelings and frustrations, and probably did stop me developing the bad habits my family were concerned about.

In order to deal with the strain on family relationships we tried family counselling, but this rarely worked well as I couldn't keep up with the conversations or express myself adequately in the sessions because it took time for me to formulate my thoughts. What was helpful to me was recording some of my own therapy sessions, the aim being that I should listen to them during the week and remind myself of what I and the therapist discussed. Although in practice this rarely happened, the tapes were useful as I would play them to my family. I found this significantly helpful as it allowed them to hear the feelings and the thoughts I found so difficult to express at the best of times, let alone in a group setting.

Chapter 9

Going it alone

Since the accident I had felt desperately alone. I knew (and know) that my family love me, but they were family, so in a way it didn't count. I did have a few years, between 1997 and 2000, when I thought I might get married. I had been going out with a doctor friend of my sister's. He is a very kind man. He visited me in America, and fixed my chair that night in college. Certain friends and relations who had shown such amazing sympathy early on developed a little of the green-eyed monster, wondering how a brain-damaged girl like me could bag such an eligible bachelor. After all, he was a doctor from a distinguished Sri Lankan family. Thankfully, I was oblivious to the barbed comments my family had to hear.

We had a simple relationship, which started out as just a friendship but then developed into a stronger kinship. He managed to get me out of the house. We would go into London to see a film or just eat Haagen-Dazs in Leicester Square, as I remember. He also reignited my fascination with cars and introduced me to *Top Gear*. We broke up after three years together. His family had tried to pressurise me to adopt my Sri Lankan middle name and to have a Hindu wedding. They didn't even mind if I never worked – all they wanted was a homemaker. It was a really tough decision: maybe I would never get such a good offer again. The compromise seemed small in their eyes; after all, I could still be a 'Christian' and I could call myself what I liked – it was just that he would not be a Christian, his parents would not be attending any Christian wedding, and they would call me by what was after all still my name but one I did not regularly use. Yet I knew deep down that they were asking me to take one step too far. My identity was already a mystery to me: my identity as a medic had gone by the time we broke up, and to lose my name, and in reality to deny my faith, was just too much.

I am quite confident that the relationship had to end when it did. Maybe, with hindsight, it should have ended sooner, but it was nevertheless a deep blow. I felt I was constantly being tested by God – cruelly being taken to the brink of happiness and then pulled back into despair. I sometimes wondered what I had done to deserve such a tough ride.

I had heard on more than one occasion in brain injury lectures how very hard it is for brain-injured people to have long-term relationships. Often the injury can break a relationship that was already established. I remember feeling very upset by these talks as it dawned on me that I might be alone for the whole of my life. Maybe because of the accident and my poor memory this fear was not strong enough to keep me in the wrong relationship.

I naturally struggled with the idea of being alone. Someone had comforted me by saying that if I couldn't get an academic qualification I could work, and if I couldn't work I could become a wife and mother. This appealed to me, and found a comfortable niche in my brain. It would be Plan C: I could enjoy the success of my children. Now all I needed was a man, though some of you reading may take issue with this! But my social circle was virtually non-existent. I had lost all outside interests. I had lost the skill of maintaining friends as I tended to assume that it was others' responsibility to work at the relationship, not mine. When I attended university I had had no energy to make friends, and with each year that passed the gulf between myself and the fresh-faced school leavers who were studying alongside me became more apparent.

My mother decided to look for suitable husbands in the Sri Lankan papers. Again, my sister was not happy. She thought they were all dodgy and that the process would be an exercise in humiliation, with some guy passing judgement on me primarily on the basis of what I looked like and how much money I had. The latter consideration had two aspects: initially I had no money and was therefore seen as a poor catch; later on I had too much money and my sister worried that any suitor's interest might be less than honourable. Rose also worried (she worries a lot!) that the combination of my desperation and slight social disinhibition (I could fall for someone who so much as smiled at me, and then inundate him with attention, unable to recognise when his interest had waned) would cause problems. I resented her for this – I couldn't see why she didn't just help me to achieve a little of the life she took for granted.

Having said that, finding love on the back pages of *News Lanka* was an unmitigated disaster. One respondent turned out to be a psycho alcoholic in Sri Lanka who sent ambling love letters a year after I pulled the plug. Others ran away as soon as they heard I had had an accident. I was desperate, and I kept the pressure on the family to find me a partner.

The other emotion that it is not easy for me to admit to is the extreme jealousy I felt over my sister's time. Once my sister was driving and I was with her. We argued about John coming on holiday with us. He wasn't family, and I just couldn't see why he needed to be there. Somehow I found myself opening the car door while my sister was driving on the M1 at 60 miles an hour (she drives quite slowly). She was shocked and burst into tears. This startled me, and I closed the door. When she was calmer she asked why I had done that. I figured that I wasn't getting my point across and that they would be better off without me. It was her crying that must have touched some deep part of me and changed my rigid thought process. My psychologist told my family that it was blackmail and that I should be ignored.

The family took the psychologist's advice, and as I remember we went on holiday anyway, with John in tow. We were staying in Knaresborough in North Yorkshire. We visited Old Mother Shipton's Cave and punted along the river Nidd. It was a good break. I had tolerated John as a necessary evil, but come Sunday evening it was time for Rose and John to return to London to start college. I was not impressed. It was a clear sign to me that I was not Rose's number one priority. John was – and worse than that, I was left with just my two ageing parents for company, bringing into sharp relief my loneliness. I went into a fury as soon as they had gone. My parents were beside themselves, and within 24 hours Rose was back in Yorkshire for an extra week. She tells me that in the three hours it took her to drive back to Yorkshire she wondered how she should respond to me. She felt angry with me for what appeared to be bullying tactics, and was feeling anxious for my parents who felt like they were being punished for something that was not their fault. She finally decided just to come and find me in my bedroom and give me a kiss on the cheek.

Rose and I have always been close, but the accident put a huge strain on our friendship that is only recovering some ten years later. The accident had made us shift roles – I became more childlike, while Rose suddenly had to grow and mature. My immature friendships foundered (the first year of college is an odd time, with everyone displaying a façade and vying to gain the biggest circle of friends, like stags in the rutting season). I soon discovered, to my cost, that the friendships hadn't been tested and were often not well rooted. Developing deep friendships is a skill that still eludes me. However, I am grateful for the few medical school friends who have tried to keep me in mind though our paths are now so different. At the same time, my accident had consolidated Rose's friendships.

Her new-found confidence also made her more sociable, while I had become socially inept.

All this hurt, and Rose really embodied my losses. I couldn't understand why my life was so lonely and different. I can honestly say that I do not believe I was jealous of Rose, as many psychologists assumed. That is not to say my actions could not have been seen as fits of jealousy. As far I was concerned, she had very little understanding of my losses and seemed to be parading her healthy, happy life. I became quite egocentric, wanting my family to make my needs, my wishes, their all-consuming desire 24 hours a day and seven days a week. I hated it when she met up with friends, even if I was invited. I wanted her all to myself, and hated anything or anyone who deflected her attention from me. Rose had been told by my psychologist to spend quality time with me. I enjoyed this time, but we both felt that to a degree it was an artificial situation, and I would accuse her of not actually wanting to be with me. She admitted that some of the time this was indeed the case.

Rose was all too aware of the losses I had suffered, and had felt extremely guilty about my struggles, even during our childhood. But she found the idea of sibling jealousy, of my being jealous of her, really difficult to handle. She could sense her own feelings of bitterness towards me bubbling up in her, and she didn't want to feel that. She tells me that within a few weeks of the accident she had made a conscious decision that she would not move far from home so that she could be with me, and then within a few months had decided she would marry John. She said it was better for her to deal with my feelings of anger than to give up John and resent me. The reality was that my sister was true to her word. She never moved further than fifteen miles away, choosing jobs so she could stay close by our family home. She and John never hugged or kissed in front of me. For many years she felt she was walking a tightrope, waiting for the day when I was more settled and my attentions would drift from her, and each failure in my plans or relationships filled her with dread.

In 2005, she tells me, we were sitting on her sofa and I told her she really needed to have children. She tearfully admitted that she wanted to, but needed to see me settled, and was scared that it would make me feel more alone, and even jealous. I cried and said how having a little niece or nephew would be the best thing that I could wish for, and how I wanted my sister to get on with her life too. We hugged and kissed, that strong bond between us finally resurfacing after a decade or more of attack. A few days later, when my sister thanked me for my words of that night, it became apparent to her that I could not remember what we had talked about. Although I had forgotten the conversation, I know my feelings have never been more true.

Rose admits that it has taken a very long time for her to really understand the extent of my losses, to cut me some slack and go with the flow of my rubbish memory, and to reduce the amount of nagging. In a funny way, writing this book has been a help. Recently I discovered quite by accident that I had been driving my car for more than six months with no insurance. The car was my responsibility. I had wanted a new car, and insisted that I was capable of making the arrangements myself. My family checking up on my work was something I could not handle; I did not want to be treated like a child, hence the delay in picking up the error. I was so scared by my oversight that I couldn't even produce my usual defensive explanations. I needed Rose's help, and was prepared for her to lay into me completely. She didn't. She made the calls and arranged the insurance; she even said we were fortunate that I had spotted it before an accident had happened. After 11 years, she says she has finally realised that shouting at me over something like this would be as pointless as asking someone in a wheelchair why they were not using the stairs.

The depression, the anger, the poor memory were all to do with my brain injury. They conspired with my general loss of role and identity to make me extremely lonely, and out of this loneliness rose the darker emotions of resentment and jealousy. My bad memory unfortunately did not stop these feelings lingering even if they were groundless. My mother is convinced that it was prayer and good therapy that were able to stop these negative feelings establishing themselves in my life and changing the course of my recovery. Now I can honestly say I find it hard to generate and harbour these negative feelings, maybe in part because we, as a family, are all moving on and learning from our mistakes.

Chapter 10

My day in court?

In 2002 the case seemed to be drawing to its conclusion. It was odd to think that when my family first obtained legal advice regarding my accident we nearly got nowhere. We went to a London-based firm recommended by one of my medical school friends whose father was a lawyer. We were trying to say that I should never have been given the particular anaesthetic I had received, as the product literature said 'use with caution in asthmatics' and I was mildly asthmatic. We were focusing on the wrong thing, asking the wrong question. The lawyers said we didn't have a case, and the solicitor advised my family not to antagonise the NHS. This seemed a harsh statement, given all that I had been through, but it was nonetheless fair – we needed everyone to help us, and the last thing we wanted to do was to come across as belligerent troublemakers. After all, as I have said before, the NHS and I were old friends.

A year later my family sought the help of a local lawyer in Watford. My parents still had the memories of the nurse grabbing them in the corridor and whispering in their ear for them to get a lawyer, and all those ambulance chasers seeking them out. They knew something had happened, and they needed to know what; no one had given them a clear explanation. For at least four or even five years after my accident we really had no idea of the train of events leading to my accident. Friends and family would ask, and we would say there had been a medical accident, but in an odd way the fact that we had not shown that the hospital was at fault worked against us. People could think we might be making it up, and as a by-product this made my experiences and my brain injury less true. I do believe the settlement has validated my experiences, at least to me. Now if I am tempted to think that there is nothing really wrong with me, I am swiftly reminded that hospitals don't just give their money away, at least not to their patients.

The second set of lawyers realised that something was amiss in the anaesthetic room records. As the significance of the accident and the damages that might be involved in my case became apparent, it moved up the hierarchy of solicitors in the firm. Even though I was merely a student at the time of my accident, my career path, and hence the earning potential I had lost, was pretty easy to track. Ironically, my own sister represented the life I could have had, not just in my eyes but now also in those of the court.

The case was set for October 2002. After nearly seven years, we had a date for a hearing at the High Court, housed in the gothic surrounds of the Royal Courts of Justice in London. In the late summer we all went in to meet the silk barrister in his chambers in the Middle Temple behind Fleet Street. He was young, probably in his forties, and he seemed to have received his training both at the Bar and at RADA. He was convinced that the hospital would settle out of court, but seemed excited at the idea of asking for at least a million pounds in damages if they did decide to show up. I was shocked. The legal system is odd. Like medicine, you are very young when you go into it, and many of the people who do enter the profession seem to have brilliant, easily distracted minds. Most medics think of themselves as amateur sleuths, and then probably get a little bored when they have figured out what is wrong with you. I think some lawyers are frustrated actors, and the courtroom serves as their stage, with justice a helpful by-product.

The barrister was right. Two weeks before the date, the hospital's lawyers informed my lawyers that they would settle out of court, for a lot less than the one million pounds but nonetheless a six-figure sum. We accepted. I was not keen to go to court, as by all accounts the other side had spent seven years and three sets of lawyers to get out of admitting responsibility, and I am sure they would have taken me to pieces regardless of all I had been through. My solicitors were concerned that I might even fail to admit to the problems I faced, and underplay my deficits.

There are two parts to a negligence claim: first you have to show that there was a lack of care, and secondly that it was this lack of care that led to the losses you have suffered. The other side might try to show that the losses you have suffered are not significant, or that they are not a direct consequence of the event but happened because you were already a waste of space! I know some of my friends from rehab have had to endure this bitter experience of court proceedings.

Mum was adamant that as few people as possible should know about the award. It was enough to know what had actually happened; the pieces all seemed to fit now. She felt that many would see the award more as a lottery win or windfall (and therefore feel jealous of me) than as a recompense for all I had endured, and my only source of income for the rest of my life. We were obviously pleased with the settlement, but there was no party or celebration. In a strange way I was going to miss meeting with my solicitor and expert witnesses. I liked them a lot and it made me feel important to know that all this work and effort was for me.

I feel incredibly lucky to have received a payout. With my award I bought my two-bedroomed flat and started on a vocational training programme for brain-injured patients.

I have met numerous people who have suffered injuries from drink drivers and the like, where the offender is never caught or the case is never brought to trial, yet the injured person has to live with the consequences. Some suffer injury through their own folly, and of course there are those who suffer brain injury because of sheer bad luck or bad genes, having suffered strokes and the like. Instead of receiving compensation, they watch their earning ability and finances crumble, with very little support to hand. The award has not given back to me the life I had hoped to be living, but it has taken much of the burden from me and my family, and that is a real blessing for which I am thankful.

My sister told me I was 'lucky' not to be a member of the medical profession, having to face decades of hard slog in a crumbling NHS. This was of little comfort to me. Whatever is said and done, deep down most medics eat, breathe and sleep medicine. It is the only thing they know to talk about, and though some medics I have met are consummate whingers, complaining about NHS bureaucracy and ungrateful patients, I am always aware that they seem to actually love their jobs. I desperately wanted to taste both the good and the bad of medicine. To choose to give up something is one thing, but to have it wrenched from your grasp leaves you with a deep ache that is indescribable. One thing was certain: however big my award, it would never allow me to be the medic I had so badly wanted to be.

My award has not given me my memory back either, but it has allowed me to live semi-independently, in a home of my choosing. I didn't have to do paid work, but at the time of receiving the award that wasn't something I was ready to give up. I see very little of the money I have. My sister deals with all my household bills, and I receive a monthly allowance. Initially when I got the flat I tried to handle my own finances, but it was a disaster. I bought impulsively, especially when I became a career girl in Westminster and had access to Marylebone High Street. I would overspend, and my direct debits for amenities would not be honoured. I had my telephone line cut off numerous times. I somehow managed to set myself up with three separate internet dial-up accounts, and I was perpetually overdrawn. My sister reminds me that I once bought four copies of Anastacia's CD on Amazon. She only knows because I gave her a copy and then asked a week later if she would like a copy. She also found further copies in my flat.

One of the best things I ever did was to get rid of my credit card. I have only one account that I handle now. My sister is always really upset at the overdraft charges I keep having to pay, and regularly brings this to my attention. She checks all my statements, which come once a week, and I have to explain my spending. I have a real problem with internet and television shopping. My boredom and the ease of buying at the click of a button mean that I can acquire five or six purchases in a day. I often don't remember what it is I have bought. I took to putting post-it notes all over my TV and computer with 'Don't buy anything' written in big bold letters, and though this would work for a week or two, I could easily go back to my bad habits if the notes fell off or were removed during a well-needed house clean.

The nagging from Rose and Mum does seem to have worked a little, as I am really trying to cut down. For those purchases that do make it through the net, Rose makes me tell her from my bank statement what it is I have bought. If I cannot remember then those items get returned unopened the day after they arrive. I know my spending like this is foolish and wasteful – anyone could walk away with my purchases and I wouldn't even know – but rational behaviour and impulsivity are not normally bedfellows. Often Rose and I have flaming rows. I tell her I want to sack her and I will find someone else less irritating. She generally retorts with: 'You can't sack me; you don't pay me. Anyway, I quit.' But as my solicitor has rightly highlighted, I have to weigh up my sister's nagging with the fact that she is cheap, charging nothing for sorting out my affairs.

Chapter 11

Vocational training

In 2003 I took a year out of my pharmacology and nutrition degree at Luton University. I was finding even this course tough going. I was living in university accommodation, sharing a flat with three other girls. Rose and John were living in Harpenden, which is the neighbouring town to Luton. They visited most days and helped me with my projects. They knew I felt lonely, and took me to their home for dinner, or we went out to eat. On Friday afternoons I would eagerly head back to my parents' house for the weekend.

My flatmates were a good few years younger than me, and the gap formed an instant barrier for them. Their vitality scared me and I got irritated by their noisy, careless behaviour. I could not concentrate on my work with their incessant chatter and music that penetrated the paper-thin walls. We had a communal kitchen, and once upon a time, before my accident, I could spend all day in such a kitchen chatting and joking. Now I scurried in when I thought the room would be empty so as to have the least chance of bumping into my boisterous flatmates. I had made a few friends on my course, but never went out with them in the evenings. I valued Rose and John's visits, and I persuaded myself that I had a life outside university. After all, I had done the communal living thing before; my spending time with my family was through choice, not necessity.

My award came at just the right time. I had wanted to go to one of the American rehab units, such as the Rusk Institute in New York. Obviously I had not considered where I would stay, whether I would get lonely or even if I might find it tough going. All I knew was that New York was great and I could live like a New Yorker. Now I finally had the resources to enrol on a vocational training programme for brain-injured people in London. It would give me a chance to take a break from studying and to see if work would turn out to be a better option for me. Thankfully, a vocational training programme had opened in London in 2001, which provided a workable alternative to my ill-thought-out plan of living in New York. I would have to travel into the Rehab UK centre at London Bridge. I was recovering from another bout of depression and anxiety, and this kind of journey did not make me feel any more relaxed. Looking back, Rusk was probably rather too fanciful!

After the initial reluctance, I started enjoying the daily train journeys into the city. As I stared out of the window, the dark gloominess of winter was replaced by the warmth of bright spring days; my depression was lifting. I met many other brain-injured people, some with serious physical disabilities and some with mainly cognitive dysfunction, like me. Most were my age or a little younger; many had suffered their injuries within the past few years if not months. I was unusual in that my accident had been so many years ago.

It is interesting to note that all of us were (and still are) single. Maybe those lecturers' sombre judgements were right. It was important for me to meet others in a similar situation to my own – well-looking in spite of significant brain injury, the so-called walking wounded. I found it harder to relate to people with obvious physical problems. I didn't believe I was like them, and sometimes I felt a fraud, believing there was nothing wrong with me as I looked so well. I made very good friends at rehab. We shared our experiences, both good and bad. For example, we discussed our feelings of anger and frustration, so I could tell that my experiences were not unique.

We learnt how to complete our CVs, and how to speak positively about our brain injury. We learnt computer skills and I gained a CLaIT qualification (computer literacy and information technology). I have always loved computers and technology – as a child I was much happier taking apart my dad's calculator or the family computer than feeding my dollies invisible tea and scones. After my accident this inclination was still there, but it became apparent to my family over the years that my skills were not as sharp as I believed them to be, and I struggled to learn new things.

I wrote an article for Rehab UK's *Renew* magazine, describing my life as a medical student and then after the accident. Maybe I needed to find some different subject matter to write about. Nonetheless, I was pleased with my achievement and to see my words in print.

I know that some people who have brain injury hate the idea of meeting with other brain-injured people, preferring to get back into the 'real world' again, and not be defined by their injury. There was a time when I only defined myself as a medical student. It has taken me ten years to come to terms with the fact that my brain injury is now the main thing that defines me, regardless of whether or not I like it. Some of my friends even consider the date of their injury as the day when they were 'born again', and if asked when their birthday is will actually give you two dates. I am not like that, but what happened to me has undoubtedly changed me, and I now acknowledge that I am a different person because of it. I have other friends who have suffered traumatic brain injury and who never went through extensive rehab programmes as I did. They have had to learn to sink or swim. Thankfully, they seem to be swimming, but it is a hard slog and I really don't know for sure that I wouldn't have sunk if left to my own devices.

The social bonding that happens when you go to a rehab unit can be powerful, and was probably the single most important thing that I benefited from. You start to develop skills like social interaction in a safe and cosseted environment, and this can be incredibly valuable. It is only really since attending rehab that I have had a social life. We met in the evenings and at weekends. Our lives had regained a refreshing normality: chatting on the phone and actively stating preferences and choices as to which film to watch or which restaurant to go to, momentarily shedding the shackles of disability, at least in our own heads.

Some of the people at the centre had been sponsored by their employers, while others had got funding through Jobcentre Plus. A few, like me, funded our rehabilitation privately, through awards and the like. I felt encouraged by the fact that some people with brain injury were making it back into variations of their old jobs, and many were getting into paid work – usually in the technical and administration fields. I worked hard, and passed swiftly through the different levels of the training programme, so that I was soon ready to organise some administration-based voluntary work. For people like me, and possibly for others without head injury, voluntary work is a fantastic way of gaining the experience that employers want when looking at candidates for salaried posts.

I found a work placement at a diabetes charity in London. It was basic administration, assisting the deputy editor of their monthly children's magazine. My role was to be an agony aunt-like character called Freddy the Frog. I had to answer kids' queries on diabetes (my bit of medical knowledge helped a lot with this), and pick competition winners. I found the job very rewarding and fun. I worked from 9 am till 3 pm two days a week, and I usually left feeling exhausted but happy. I did this job for five months, and I loved it.

My family were keen that I stay on and asked if there were any paid positions. But I was again on a high, puffed up by my success and stubborn as a mule. I decided to go back to Luton and finish that degree. My dream of getting an academic qualification was still alive and well. I had an impressive practical study project lined up, seeing whether food advertising altered the shopping choices that people made before these adverts became a part of daily viewing on the television and after. I think it would have been cool to actually do this study. But I had forgotten the struggles I had had with the BSc timetable, let alone with functioning as a college student. Within two months I had decided to leave Luton. However, with the credits I had gained in my first year I achieved a Higher National Certificate (HNC) in Pharmacology with Nutrition. I have to get the whole title in, as it's so important to me now – a brain-injured person who succeeded in getting an academic qualification. Even as I type, I am giving myself a smug little pat on the back!

I had actually graduated from Rehab UK when I went back to my degree, so I attended my graduation ceremony at City Hall, the home of our then mayor, Red Ken. It was a bitter January day, with the wind swirling and howling manically and giving the impression that City Hall had assumed its odd shape by physically resisting being blown into the Thames by the force of the gale. I had not attended a graduation from Luton, having left there early, so the Rehab UK graduation was very special. It was my first and possibly my last graduation ceremony. The venue was excellent. The security was intense, but this almost made you feel like exclusive VIP guests. The graduation took place in what was probably one of the larger meeting rooms. We, the graduates, and our families sat facing our panel of smiling therapists, behind them London's beautiful, if slightly oppressive, skyline. There is something very significant in knowing that you have accomplished a goal against the odds. I received my CLaIT certificate that day. It was not mere pieces of paper we were given, but recognition of our achievements.

My family had a chance to meet my friends and their families. Rose was struck by how sad and futile all the stories were, and how many of the families had many other problems to deal with on top of their loved ones' head injuries. She felt that they all looked happy but very tired, and uncertain for their loved ones' futures – anxiety masked by hopeful pleasant smiles, as she put it. As some of the course organisers and the charity's patron gave their speeches, the slightest flicker of recognition of what we had been through and achieved, even though given by people who themselves were not brain-injured, was gratefully received, and quickly brought tears to the eyes of our relatives and loved ones.

My mother proudly hung my certificates on her study wall alongside my music exam certificates and my sister's medical qualifications. Even though I fight with Mum, I have to acknowledge that she went out of her way to make me feel an equal. When my sister became a member of the Royal College of Physicians she had some portrait pictures done. My mother always felt her wall was lopsided with just my sister's photos hanging there, so she arranged to have some formal portraits done of me too, to hang alongside my sister's.

I finally put to rest the idea of being an academic. I was too old anyway, having just had my thirtieth birthday. It was time I went out into the job market. Rehab UK agreed to take me back and support me while I looked for another job. My boss at Diabetes UK had moved on and they had filled my post with a paid employee, so I had to start again from square one, looking for more voluntary work or, even better, a paid job.

I had started doing a few hours' voluntary work in basic administration for two local charities, to keep up my skills. I decided that I would apply for part-time jobs in administration. I was so motivated that I even enrolled on an evening course to gain my ECDL (European Computer Driving Licence). My dad and I did this course together. We practised on the computer in the evenings and visited the library. I think he was a little peeved when I got a higher mark than him.

I started my search while at Rehab UK, and continued when I returned home at the end of each day. I usually got home at around five, and after my daily dose of *Neighbours* I would eat and then browse through the local paper and through the *Metro* that I had picked up on my journey home from London. I had been taught to look for 'two tick' organisations, which actively supported disabled employees. I came across a job that was for only 18 hours per week, displayed the two ticks and was based at one of Westminster Council's offices in Baker Street. I had never worked more than four or six hours a week in my voluntary jobs so 18 hours was a big jump, but on the other hand it was well below the forty hours that full-timers worked. I could see no reason why I shouldn't be able to manage. It seemed perfect, and I applied. I did not hear from them for about a month, but in spite of this I pretended in my head that I had been invited for an interview and would make my job coaches give me mock interviews. I had gone through numerous university interviews and felt certain that job interviews could not be as hard as those, but I was taking no chances.

In the following weeks I did get shortlisted for an interview for the Baker Street job. I was ecstatic and at the same time scared, as all this real vocational stuff was so new to me. I attended my interview feeling nervous and apprehensive. I was interviewed by two people, the manager and his deputy. It was fairly laid back, and I was relieved that all those months of working and studying seemed to have come to fruition. I think that when they saw what an extensive educational background I had, and also how I was trying to overcome my disability, my prospective employers must have felt sorry for me and wanted to give me an opportunity to prove myself.

I completed the interview and then met up with my parents. My mum was attending Moorfields Eye Hospital, as her vision had been affected by the neurosarcoid she had developed the year after my accident. My dad was driving us back from Moorfields when the manager who had interviewed me rang my mobile. It took a few rings before I had composed myself enough to hear their verdict. The manager asked how I would feel if he offered me the job. I was overjoyed to say the least, and could have whooped with joy. Instead, I accepted with as much restraint as I could muster. This was probably the second biggest achievement I have made so far, the first being recovering from my accident in the first place.

We celebrated by going for a sumptuous dinner at the new and extremely expensive Grove Hotel in Hertfordshire. Dinner was on me. I finally had a respectable answer to that fundamental, if not highly impertinent, question that is the nub of many social interactions: 'What do you do?', or all too often in my case, 'Are you a doctor too?' This question had stumped me for nearly a decade. Whenever it was asked I would stare furtively at my family, desperate for them to take over. After all, Joe Public didn't need to know my whole life history and hadn't asked to hear it, but each time I hummed and hahhed it was as though I was either a complete layabout or some sort of cretin. Now I had my answer: 'Gosh no, I am definitely not a doctor. I work in admin!'

I had two weeks in which to say goodbye to my friends at the two voluntary jobs I was in. I got some lovely cards and well-wishes. I was about to become a fully paid-up city commuter, working nine to five (well, almost) – what a way to make a living! But first, some shopping. I needed a new wardrobe, possibly some nice skirts and matching jackets. Oh, and I would need a new pair of shoes, or maybe two.

Chapter 12

Working girl

I woke up keen and eager to start my first day at Westminster Council. It was late October. I was going to be based in Marylebone Road, at Council House, an imposing Georgian building with huge stone lions guarding the steps up to the entrance. (At Christmas time they had the tallest tree you have ever seen standing in the foyer. That year it was decked in pretty little scarlet bows, and it made me feel like I was in New York – my second favourite city.)

It would be a fairly easy trip in to work, the Metropolitan underground line taking me the entire way. In all it would take 40 minutes by train plus a five-minute walk at either end. I really enjoyed my commute into work. Watford is at the end of the Metropolitan line so I was always guaranteed a crisp fresh copy of the free daily paper, the *Metro*, and a seat from which I could happily observe my fellow commuters. Most of these seemed distinctly underwhelmed by the prospect of starting another week's work. For my part, I was thrilled to be working at last, and was the irritatingly happy member of the carriage.

I enjoyed people-watching, and I was (and still am) always mystified by ladies who got on the train looking as if they had just stepped out of the shower, with still-damp combed-back hair, and during the course of the journey managed to groom themselves, applying make-up and even mascara, so as to arrive at their destination immaculate and unflustered; I was certainly not one of those girls! Usually I would read the *Metro* or whatever book I was enjoying at the time, and stumble into and out of the carriage with as much elegance as a baby rhino.

By the end of my journey I had gleaned the news headlines and concocted elaborate stories in my head about the passengers who were sitting in front of me on that occasion.

Once at Baker Street, I would sit and sip a hot chocolate in one of the many cafés. I loved London and I loved this bit of London. After my drink I would walk to the library next door to the Council House so that I could glance at a few titles. It never occurred to me to become a member and go on to borrow and read these titles. I don't really know why I was looking, as my memory was so poor that I would be unable to remember the names anyway, but it helped to while away a few minutes. I did not start work until ten o'clock but I always arrived well before then.

I would come into the building and breezily show my pass to the security man. I was in a big office on the first floor. I even had my name on the door: Antoinette Anthony-Pillai – assistant administrator. I was in a large high-ceilinged room, probably quite elegant in its time but now furnished with standard-issue public sector short-pile brown carpet, functional grey metal cupboards and angular tables. I shared the room with my boss, who had interviewed me, and two other women.

Usually when I got into the office I would greet my colleagues and make a coffee, then sit down to commence my day's work. Every job I did felt like I was doing something new and fresh, not really remembering where I had left off previously. The upside to my memory loss is that I am seldom annoyed with others for long as I forget incidents, and holding and maintaining grudges is something I find quite difficult to do. Unlike when I was at medical school, where I battled with my memory problems and my depression, my mood was actually very good now and I had no idea if I was doing anything wrong. If my colleagues were irritated or annoyed by me, I didn't register it. Most things just 'washed over me'. All four of us would go out for lunch, sometimes joined by the technical wizards who worked alongside us carrying out the computer sessions that my office organised. I had to make stationery orders, generate invoices and file receipts from local primary schools that used our computer services.

We all seemed to get on so well, texting each other jokes and generally having a laugh in those early days. I couldn't believe my luck, landing such a nice job with such nice people. I would check my email when the day was quieter, and encourage friends and family to email me so that I didn't feel like a Norma no-mates. I bought a little rose plant for my table. I had grown my nails and they were perfectly manicured. I had my Rehab UK file with notes and prompts by the side of my table, but it didn't seem that I really needed them. I had this admin thing in the bag.

In late December my boss informed me that they would be extending my probation and had secured funding for extra help from Rehab UK, via Jobcentre Plus, to help me with strategies for work. I was thrilled and told my family the news: 'See, they really want to help me. They must really like me.' My mother was not so convinced.

That was the Christmas when my father decided to leave us. Maybe my enthusiasm allowed him to finally convince himself that his paternal duties were completed. He had coped with my accident by maintaining a significant emotional distance from all of us. I believe that after the accident his admiration for me changed to a feeling of pity. I know that my becoming ill, followed by my mum's significant illness, was not consistent with a life he wanted or could handle. He knew I needed him around if I was to find a Sri Lankan husband, since prospective Asian mothers-in-law would not be very impressed by the daughter of divorced parents. After all, what would it say about the girl's morals and commitment? But doing the right thing just because you feel sorry for someone is an onerous task, and in 2004 my father decided he had to start looking out for himself. He has made no contact with any of us since then, and we are told that he now lives in Sri Lanka. I still love him to bits and hope he is well. It is odd, because unlike with Mum and Rose I never really fought with my dad. His leaving was a surprise to me, but we all responded to it matter-of-factly. To have done anything else would have been too emotionally draining, I suppose. Also, I have to admit that, in a funny way, my father leaving took some of the pressure off looking through all those personal ads in the paper.

In February, which is never a good month for me, I was given the boot. My sister was furious. My description of how I was doing and their actions just didn't match up. She called up my trade union representative, and came with me to meet with my boss. We finally managed to convince the human resources department that they should try to redeploy me in line with their duties under the Disability Discrimination Act. My sister said it was odd to see how desperate and traumatised my boss appeared. He couldn't bear to look at us. He kept saying he knew it was not my fault, but he just wanted me out of his office. They had compiled a huge file documenting all the errors I had made, with both money and stationery orders, and how on a few occasions I had simply forgotten to come in to work. All I could say through my tears was, 'Well, if you don't want me then I don't want to be here.'

I went down and collected my plant, but I forgot my prompt file (which unfortunately then got binned). My mum and sister had not had time to think about what would happen if this job did not work out. For the past year I had done administration work and had done it quite well in my voluntary posts – this is not just my analysis, but based on my references. If this job went, they were certain that I would slip into a depression, and they had no idea what the options were. The redeployment was as much for my family as for me; they needed the time to get their thoughts together and to help me to plan. I did slip into depression anyway. It suddenly dawned on me that I wasn't able to do a job I considered basic – so what was I good for? It took nearly five months to get me redeployed. In the meantime I returned to my voluntary jobs. My friends there welcomed me back with a much-appreciated hug.

I have to say that one lesson I have learned is that it is important to consider joining a trade union when you start work. The Disability Discrimination Act puts in place safeguards for disabled employees, but that does not stop even well-meaning 'two tick' employers from trying to shove a disabled employee out on the quiet. Many of my friends who have also lost their jobs have just left and then sunk into a depression, not knowing anything about the duties of the employer to support them in their work. This is where a trade union representative can help, and organisations such as the Disability Rights Commission are willing to advise if you don't have trade union representation.

The man in human resources was really kind. Again it was clear that he felt very sorry for me, and he worked hard to see what other job they could find for me within the council. They made sure they did everything fairly and by the book, and decided to get a formal report of my abilities from Dr Oddy, who was now based at the Brain Rehabilitation Trust in Surrey. It was good to see him again after nearly nine years. I couldn't really see what I had done wrong, and I reminded him that my references from voluntary work were good and that my sister was convinced that this was all due to my not being used to the nuances of a working environment, rather than anything to do with my memory. She believed I just needed more time to learn the different elements of the role, and for the role to be honed a little. I nodded in agreement.

Finally my employer, my sister and my trade union representative managed to get me redeployed to work as a library assistant at St John's Wood Library. I met the manager, who knew about my brain injury and was keen to support me so long as I managed to perform in my interview. During the interview process I was made to read a story to four slightly overweight middle-aged men and women, pretending they were five-years-old – a challenge for anyone to do with a straight face. Anyway, they accepted me. St John's Wood is a beautiful area to work in. It has slightly nicer coffee shops than Baker Street and some fantastic independent art shops and galleries that became my haunts. What was more, I would be working with what have become among my favourite things in the world: books. My other favourite thing is stationery, as my former boss was all too well aware!

Chapter 13

Truth hurts

I commenced my job at St John's Wood Library, and I loved it. I was doing 18 hours a week. I was to work as a library assistant behind the front desk, checking in and checking out books, DVDs, videos and music. I had learnt a few lessons from the singes I had sustained in my last job. I was a little more wary of having a joke and a laugh with my workmates and decided that the priority was to get my work done and to get through the probation. I knew nothing was guaranteed until I had managed to survive those few months.

When I first started at St John's Wood I was sent on an introductory day that the libraries run, so that I could be familiarised with the 14 or so libraries that came under Westminster Council. One of the stops on the tour was at Victoria Music Library. Here I was taken down to the deepest, darkest recesses of the basement to see some original manuscripts from composers such as Haydn and Tchaikovsky. To say I was bowled over is putting it mildly! To see these great individuals' writing on original manuscript sheets, complete with blotting splodges, was one of the best moments in my life so far.

The St John's Wood Library is small, but really very busy. Working behind the till was hard. The residents of the area must have been use to snapping their fingers and getting things done in a split second. The CD and DVD prices were all individualised on a sheet of paper, and local residents could get special discounts if they brought in their discount cards. Many tried to get discounts without their cards, and to say that they could be intimidating is an understatement.

Once a lady walked in, and after she had been in the queue for a while, waiting for me to serve her, I could hear her tutting and sighing as she shifted her weight from one hip to the other. She was finally at the front of the queue.

'Can you move any slower?' she asked in an irritated tone. 'My car is on a double yellow line and I need to get out of here. I have never seen such awful service.'

I stared at my sheet of paper with the DVD prices on it. 'It's not my fault if you chose to park illegally,' I said, not even attempting to look up.

I was so proud of myself. It was the first time in ages that I had 'given as good as I got'. I collected her money in exchange for her DVD and she attempted to swan out, but I had clearly ruffled her feathers.

'Antoinette, can I speak to you?' It was my supervisor; she had been watching our little exchange. 'You mustn't let the customers wind you up. You should have just not answered back.' I couldn't tell if she was annoyed or impressed, but it didn't matter – I was very pleased with myself and could not wait to tell Mum and Rose.

Part of my role was to be an assistant with the under-fives' group. I would have to do songs with dances, learn nursery rhymes and read short stories to the toddlers. I loved this area, viewing it as training for the imminent arrival of my niece, and it also took me back to my own childhood. The under-fives were a great laugh. Once I had a group of Muslim children, and one made me smile by asking me secretively, 'Would you like to see my hair?' and then slowly pulling back her headscarf, exclaiming with delight: 'See, I have hair too!'

I seemed to get favourable feedback from my boss, though she did complain that I was not spontaneous enough and would need prompting to go on to another song. I took her criticism seriously, but I believed that the children liked me, and that was all that really counted. It was a fantastic boost to my self-esteem. Even now I find myself humming 'The wheels on the bus go round and round, round and round ...' in idle moments. This was indeed superb preparation for my new niece, as once she could hold her head up unaided I was quick to teach her all the songs and rhymes I knew. I brought home numerous pregnancy books for Rose so that she would be up to speed on all the latest child-rearing techniques, and I would do my own bit of research on the best and most popular baby reads for my niece. After all, I didn't want her to fall behind and get picked on by the other toddlers at her nursery! She loves books now (at the grand old age of 20 months, at the time of writing), and I like to think that I helped nurture some of that early fascination.

So back to my story. I had to learn the entire library procedures regarding loaning out books and multimedia material (including DVDs and videos, along with music CDs), and also had to take payment for these and be able to operate the till well and account for every transaction. The council could not afford any more input from Rehab UK or other support services, so Dr Oddy introduced me to Dr Sherrie Baehr, who would help and support me at work. I was again struggling to keep up. I met with Dr Baehr weekly and she spoke regularly to my boss and visited me at work. She gave me strategies and told me to drink plenty of water to counter the headaches I was again experiencing. I made numerous mistakes with money and with the filing of books, but I was convinced that I had done everything properly. When I was pulled up I agreed I was in the wrong, but couldn't really understand what the fuss was about. So I gave back 50p and not 5p, and I filed 'n' before 'm' – hardly worth getting over-excited about!

I can't remember the exact day. All I know is that it was cold and I lay snuggled under my duvet. The phone rang. I rolled over and picked up the receiver from my bedside table.

'Hello, can I speak to Antoinette?'

'Yes, speaking'

'Antoinette, we were expecting you at work this morning at nine o'clock.'

I looked at my clock. It was 9.15. I fumbled for an answer. I didn't have one. 'I am so sorry. I will be there in the next half an hour.' The caller hung up.

I rang my mum in a state of panic.

'Go and get ready. I will call Rose.'

Ten minutes later there was a knock at the door, and my sister stood there. It was the first week of her maternity leave and she was heavily pregnant, wearing a ski jacket that would only fasten at the top, above the expanse of her tummy. Mum had told her not to have a go at me. I must have looked stressed. My hair was still uncombed and I was struggling to get my boots on.

'What are you going to do?'

'I am just about to run and get the train.'

'Anto, it will take you at least an hour to get in.'

'What else can I do?'

'Look, I'll drive you in – that way you've got some chance of composing yourself.'

I felt relieved. It would cut 20 minutes off the journey time. We got into the car, and before long I felt relaxed enough to give my side of the story.

'You know, they must have changed my times without telling me. I wasn't supposed to start till two today.'

'Surely you must write down your shifts?'

'Yes, I do, and I have an email printout of them too. They are all here in my diary.' I scrambled around in my handbag and proudly pulled out my small leather-bound Portable Memory. 'Look,' I said, giving her the book, with my thumb holding the pages open on the right week.

'Anto, it says 9 am here. Did you not check last night?'

'Yes. Yes, I did. I don't understand.'

The lights changed to green and we drove off again. Neither of us spoke for the rest of the journey. We turned in past the St John's Wood underground station.

'Can you drop me off here? I don't want them to see you bringing me.'

My sister reached over and kissed me on the forehead. 'Good luck, and do the best you can'.

Unfortunately, my getting the wrong time for turning up at work was not a one-off event. It happened on other occasions. I found shift work hard. Maybe there is a stubbornness in me that just cannot admit that my memory is no good, that I need to check and recheck, to use reminders and prompts, as I have been told time and time again.

Rose says that by this stage she was finally coming to terms with what was going on. My colleagues didn't understand me, and got frustrated at my asking the same stupid questions and making the same stupid mistakes time and again. The log book of errors grew, as did some not-really-necessary descriptions of how my workmates felt about me. Dr Baehr could see that I was on a hiding to nothing.

I loved the job, but this time I did not cry when they told me they were letting me go. Dr Baehr had tipped me off. I conceded defeat, and so did my sister. Rose tells me that it was only after this traumatic 15 months of my struggling to survive in the job market that she finally appreciated the full extent of my problems. She knew I loved the job, and even more so the new identity I had created for myself, and thus she was well aware that it was something I would not willingly have given up, or consciously squandered. I still don't really know what went wrong at work. I certainly was not depressed. My sister thinks that maybe I had no benchmark with which to compare how I was doing, so I assumed all was OK, whereas with my studies maybe subconsciously I could tell when I was falling behind, hence my bouts of depression during the courses.

I continue to see Dr Baehr, who somehow manages to maintain professionalism with true friendship. I had two further bouts of depression – one while between jobs and one after I finally got the sack from Westminster Council.

In December 2005 I was invited to a Christmas drinks party hosted by Dr Baehr in her Harley Street offices. I went with my mum. I like Christmas and the party season, and it was nice to get dressed up – something I loved before the accident and have started to enjoy again. I met many of Dr Baehr's other clients, some with brain injury and some with ME. It struck me that many had had to give up on their careers, and their aspirations had changed. All looked physically well but they struggled to be the useful citizens society, and they themselves, wanted them to be.

That evening I met the actress and author Jane Lapotaire. She had suffered from aneurysms in her brain, and as a result of meeting her I read her book *Time out of Mind*, about her experiences of recovery from brain injury. That was something of a turning point for me, as I started to realise that there was just a chance I could still pick up some of the pieces of what I had hoped my life would be – a chance for my existence to make some kind of impression, for my return from the dead to have some kind of meaning, at least for me if not for others. It was after this party that I decided to write down my own story.

Lastly, I just have to say (for my own record) that while I was at St John's Wood Library I met Jarvis Cocker and got his autograph for my brother-in-law who is mystifyingly keen on Jarvis's band Pulp. I also saw – wait for it – Mr Amazing, the one and only Robbie Williams! I was, and am even now, *so* in love with him. What a dream come true!

Chapter 14

Looking forward

I suppose I am now nearing the end of my written account, though it is by no means the end of the story. So maybe it is time for a little reflection, looking back on the journey so far. As I said in the beginning, it is not a journey I had envisaged or planned for my life. In some ways it has been like doing a rather dodgy crash course in diving. You are completely unfamiliar with the equipment, you hold on desperately to your guide's hand and you marvel in awe at seeing the world in which you live in a different light, only to suddenly become aware that your goggles are filling with water, your ears hurt, you are forgetting even how to breathe and you don't know how to let others know you are drowning.

In some ways it is the long mountain climb, with moments when you look back at how far you have come and smile to yourself. You can see the summit, but as you walk on you realise you have been tricked and that all that is in front of you is another impossible-looking vertical face of hard rock that you must negotiate.

As someone who has suffered both physical and cognitive ill health, I have to say the latter is harder to understand, whether you are the sufferer or the observer, and harder to compensate for. As a child I used my mind and my intellect to understand and overcome my physical health problems. When my mind was scrambled and my intellect damaged, the resources to understand and overcome my disabilities were that much harder to muster.

On 26 February 2006, 11 years and a day after my accident, my sister gave birth to my niece. Rose had a difficult birth with a nasty tear and a bad bleed. She looked extremely frail in those early days. Since having the baby, my sister seems much more chilled and less of a control freak. My niece has taken some of the gloom out of Februaries. She is a real bundle of joy, but tires me out completely after even a few minutes. I have decided that having children is probably not for me, but I am never saying never.

Rose made me godmother to her daughter. It is a role I pride myself in. I have a sense that I may never see my dreams fulfilled through my own children. I am starting to accept that even if I found the right man the risks of the pregnancy and birth might be high, given my previous surgery and bouts of depression. At one time I craved children but those feelings are no longer so strong. My god-daughter is probably the cleverest girl I have ever met, with a memory that is scarily sharp. I visit her almost daily, and on the days when I don't go to her she comes to me to play with the cats. When I visit I invariably return two seconds after leaving to collect my keys that I have forgotten to pick up. My niece, no more than a year old at the time, once saw me leaving without my keys and promptly picked them up and chased after me. She seems to like me, to love me in a way I have missed for many years now, running to greet me with sheer delight in her eyes, with a fondness disproportionate to the few hours we have spent apart. My sister is due her second baby in a few weeks' time. The due date is late March, and I know I will become a godmother again. It seems as if Rose or someone in the know has timed the births as recompense for my accidents.

My headaches are definitely better, and I am sure that drinking plenty of water and taking some regular exercise helps with this. I have found that one of my most important purchases has been a pedometer. It really encourages me to keep moving, something I found difficult for many years in spite of my athletic childhood. Of course my family do have to remind me to wear it! I am convinced that avoiding alcohol is one of the most important things for a head-injured person to do. In the beginning I did find I missed it, partly because I knew how much it was a part of my old self, but now being teetotal has become second nature.

I know I have problems with impulsive behaviour. For me that is mainly buying stuff I really don't need. I know I will probably get depressed again at some point, most likely in the winter, but hopefully I will have a bit of a break before that day comes. My GP has kindly prescribed me one week of winter sun in the Canary Islands or Ghana. Unfortunately this does not seem to come on the NHS!

I also still get angry quickly, though my all-out rages have stopped. The anger is different from argumentativeness – my family say it's like living with a firecracker, my initial response often being to snap out an answer. I know this hasn't been easy for my family, who take a little longer to forget than me, especially if I have been shouting at them in public! Over the years my mum and sister have learnt to live with my hot temper and to let it wash over them, and for this I am very grateful. For my part, as Dr Baehr has taught me, as soon as I start to feel angry or unable to express myself (which remains the primary reason for my frustration and flares of temper), I try to get out of the room straight away, and the change of scene usually calms me quickly. My family now recognise this as my way of resolving the situation, not me ignoring them.

I still find it difficult to order some areas of my life. My family know my intentions are good and do try to hand over responsibility to me, but my mistakes can be costly and time-consuming. Invariably there are frayed nerves, in spite of our best efforts. An example of this came a few months ago when I volunteered to book the tickets for a trip to Ireland but booked the wrong day, so my family had to spend many hours trying to get the dates changed at extra cost. Obviously I get annoyed and embarrassed when errors are pointed out to me, but I keep no record of my mistakes or my successes. My family reluctantly reminded me of this incident as an example for this book. It took me a little while to remember we had even been to Ireland! Even now, though I know my memory is poor, there is no part of me that questions whether I might be wrong about something. If I need to check my diary or write down a phone conversation and in the heat of the moment I forget the problems with my memory and depend on it, it is at my own cost.

My family tell me I work on an emotional level, so I get angry if I feel stressed. I see everything as brilliant if I am calm, and I send touching cards and pretty flowers, which my mum just loves. I can misconstrue someone's friendliness so that I think they are the best person ever (and in the early years I could easily mistake friendliness from a man for affection). I construe it as criticism when someone (usually my sister) questions me about something. I act impulsively, as friends and family know, firing off email and text messages to update the world on what I am doing, and probably not giving a second thought as to whether my solicitor is all that interested in the fact that I have just run two miles or am in the mood for a chocolate ice cream. I now have a cleaner, as my sister couldn't handle how I describe myself as a neat-freak and yet frequently forget to vacuum. I would try to explain that the vacuum didn't work, but the reality was that the bag needed changing and I couldn't remember where I had put the bags away.

My memory does cause me problems, mainly in my social interactions, as my concentration is poor and I switch off within minutes, even when very nice or interesting people are talking to me. But I cannot overemphasise the big plus, which is that I forget the bad stuff, especially my negative feelings, just as quickly.

In 2004 I got two goldfish, one of whom is now three years old. I like the fact that they supposedly have a worse memory than I do. In December 2006 I got two cats – who says life should be straightforward? I have managed to live in my flat for a whole year now, whereas often in the past the bouts of depression and anxiety took me back to my mother's home, as I was in no fit state to look after myself. Before last year the longest I had managed on my own at a stretch was just a few months.

Having lost my jobs in London, I worked for one week in the call centre at John Lewis, Watford. I am sure that I took the job because the room was air conditioned and when I applied it was a warm May day, and also because of the partnership discount card. Obviously these factors seemed more important to me at the time than the fact that I have no ability to remember telephone conversations, especially if an element of stress or urgency is added.

After John Lewis I decided to restart my voluntary work. I work two days a week at the Watford Citizens Advice Bureau as assistant to the manager. I do filing, shredding and posting letters, and sometimes I get to use my computer skills to do spreadsheets. I also volunteer one morning a week at a local church in Watford, linked to the one I attend in Chorleywood. Here I am in charge of doing an inventory of the books in their Book Swap scheme, having bragged about my previous library experience.

I know paid employment is unlikely to ever become a reality for me. My ideal job would be two to three hours a couple of times per week, with no noise, minimal stress and the provision for me to undertake tasks one at a time with no interruptions and at my own pace. I don't think anyone would pay me to work like that! Having said that, voluntary work has provided me with the routine I so desperately need. Thanks to it my social skills and confidence have improved hugely. I have had to develop a sense of commitment, and it has given a focus to my week. But most importantly, I feel appreciated and useful. In return I want to do the best job I can. I really would urge anyone with a brain injury to take up voluntary work, even if it ends up being just a stepping stone to something else. It is probably the single most important factor in aiding my ongoing rehabilitation.

I have never been one to speak much about my faith, and I am definitely no Ned Flanders. Maybe I am more like Tony Blair. But I know my faith has seen me through the very hard years, and will see me through what is yet to come. Christ is a definite reality in my life. I believe my family's commitment to Christ is what allowed them to show such commitment to me. Like all good and deep relationships, ours may not be perfect but they are grounded in love. As you can see, I am in no way a picture of a perfect Christian, but I know God loves me and has protected me. I would love to quote Scripture and say this verse really helped and I held on to this message, or to talk in some spiritual way, but to do so would be a lie. The truth is that I do believe the prayers of many have upheld me, especially in those times when I could not pray for myself. But more than that I think God's greatest miracle for me is to allow me to forget my feelings of anger even towards him.

On a practical note, I know that church is part of my rehabilitation. It allows me to focus on positive things. The sermons make me do a degree of healthy self-analysis. I am so pleased that church no longer brings on a migraine for me and that I can enjoy the songs, sermons and fellowship. Right now, I have decided to become a member of a church in the neighbouring town of Chorleywood. It is a little smaller and a little quieter. I miss my old church in London – I had been there since I was twelve years old, and they are my family – but the journey was just too long. Now I zip along the M25, and then enjoy serene drives through Chorleywood's country lanes.

I have two cats, Dusty and Socks, born in a trucker's yard. I got them from the animal rescue centre. The process was almost as rigorous as that for adopting a child! I wanted to have a flat cat (in other words, one that stays indoors) or else it would quickly end up a flat cat on the busy A418 that runs outside my apartment. The manager came to see my home and told me that if I wanted a house cat then I would need two so they could keep each other company. It wasn't my original plan, and double the trouble and double the fun has been very hard work for me. The animal rescue came to check on them six months after they had moved in. The manager told me they looked healthy and happy. I was so pleased – I had done that for them. My cats are great companions to me. They help me to see beyond myself, refocusing my thoughts onto their needs and comforts. They chase each other round the flat, their little bells jingling, and then exhaustedly come and crash out on my lap or in the kitchen sink. They have scratched me a couple of times and have trashed my sofa. Like I told my sister, Plan C is still active, namely I would like to get married one day, or to have a companion (human variety), but I don't feel as desperate as I did.

I try to run (though in reality it is more of a shuffle) each Saturday morning with an all-female running group. I do find winters difficult, and my mood still takes a little bashing during the months of less daylight. In this time I need to work even harder to keep myself motivated. Often my exercise routine slackens off and my weight goes up, but my spending, much to the relief of my sister, goes down. It is during this time that I teeter more precariously on the brink of depression. I have a good relationship with my local college, and try to do occasional short courses in subjects such as photography and cooking. Sometimes I have made wrong choices. Recently I booked on an advanced photography course, failing to take on board that it was aimed at people working towards a career in photography. I lasted five weeks before having to call it a day.

Now the college help me not to make inappropriate decisions. They check any application I make, knowing that I am likely to think that a course title sounds interesting and hand over my money without having any real idea of what is involved.

For the last year I have been attending a book club, which I love. We meet once a month in a local hotel. I have yet to persuade them to read one of my book choices, but there is always next month, I suppose. I often forget to read the book I am meant to read (and buy ten others from Amazon while on a high from an enjoyable book club evening), and when I do read the book of the month I have nothing more than a single word synopsis – boring or brilliant. But I have made good friends. I have started music lessons to get back into playing the piano. It is amazing how stiff my fingers have become; I used to be able to really tickle those ivories, but I have to admit that I haven't got out of my bad habit of only practising on the day of my lesson, still convincing myself that my teacher will never know. I try to do some Brain Training every day, and my brain age varies between forty and eighty years old – but I am sure that is because it doesn't register my voice.

I have got some good friends – some whom I have kept from medical school, some from rehab, some from courses, some from my social activities, and some from church. They are the most diverse group one could imagine, but they are getting to know me. They have had to adjust to the fact that I may ring up just because I am bored and fancy a milkshake, forgetting that they have young families to tend to, or may turn up at their house with a cake I have spent three hours making because I got the wrong date for a tea party.

Over the years I have developed an appreciation of the need for routine. For most people this is imposed on them through being employed or running a household. All the rehabilitation facilities I attended were very structured, because they were well aware of how important routine is. The problem was that when I was not in the rehab environment I couldn't generate a routine for myself, partly because I was often depressed but mainly because I had little understanding of how important it is for us as human beings to have structure in order to function well. I am certain that this is the reason why retirement can be such a crunch time for people who have not planned what to do with their week, once the daily commute and nine-to-five is gone. That is not to say it is not hard to keep my routine going when I do feel low. I instantly feel the need to pull back, telling myself, 'I am doing too much. I need to drop these activities and rest.' My family try desperately to persuade me to keep the activities going, even though it is counter-intuitive to me. It is a struggle.

So finally I have taken to writing up a weekly timetable. Dr Baehr has told me that actually writing things down is better than just printing off a timetable from the computer. There is something in the physical process of writing that engages different parts of the brain and helps create a stronger memory. I am sure I have been told this dozens of times over the many years of rehab I have had, but I needed to hear it again. Monday is for cleaning the fish tank, reading a book, doing some chores and having my weekly weigh-in at Weight Watchers. On Tuesdays I do voluntary work and have a piano lesson. Wednesdays I do voluntary work, and then have a well-deserved rest. Thursdays I do voluntary work. Friday is a day off. Saturdays I do my grocery shop, and on Sunday I cook for the week. I have a note on my large kitchen bin saying not to put cat litter into it but to take it to the outside bin, to stop me from stinking out the flat. I continue to see Dr Baehr – once a month now, and more if I am starting to get depressed: this usually starts with me feeling suddenly panicky or anxious.

It is twelve years since my accident. I feel I have come on in leaps and bounds. I know my life has changed in ways that I could never have imagined, and I have suffered many losses. I have gone from studying my beloved medicine – which I had seen as my destiny all those years ago – to shredding paper and filing letters, and although this does hurt (especially seeing it now written in black and white), I am doing OK. I love my jobs. I have a loving family who work hard to allow me to maintain my independence. I have a god-daughter who adores me and another god-child on the way. I have made some good friends, and I can honestly say I wouldn't change a thing. I am so thankful that, given I had to have this happen to me, I neither died nor became consumed with regret or hatred. In a way my memory loss has helped me to move on with life. I still snap at my mum, though I am trying to do this less.

I have just returned from a cultural tour of India, just my mum and me. How very Edwardian! Though the holiday completely ruined my routine, I know I have done something many would love to do but never get the chance to. I pray I will never forget the experience of entering the palace complex through the red-bricked gate house, and getting my first glimpse of the Taj Mahal emerging as a majestic apparition from the expanse of the smoggy Agra sky. Mum and I got to touch the cool marble of this awesome structure, more like a palace than a tomb, and see the intricate inlay of bright semi-precious stones enveloping this building which on first impression appears monochromic white. The highlight, according to the guide, was to see the sun setting behind the Taj Mahal, and we were duly escorted to the ideal spot. We stood in the sandy bed of the river running behind the Taj with the new, more pungent, less impressive, frankly squalid Agra all around us. Mum and I tried to skip over the pats of cow manure that dotted the ground, as well as working hard to dodge the bullock carts that ambled across the sand.

Unfortunately the pink hues of the setting sun reflecting off the majestic mausoleum never materialised as promised, owing to the low cloud. My sister could not help laughing when she heard my flat description, tinged with disappointment. She remarked on how my experiences of the Taj Mahal were in a sense symbolic of my life, in that what we thought would be the highlight, the reflected glory of the sun on the Taj, never materialised, and yet the structure was utterly captivating in its own right – more beautiful and intricate than anyone could imagine, but its beauty only fully appreciated by those who manage to see it at close range. Make sense of that if you can.

Recently I was at my sister's house. She had just returned from work with Maria, and I played with my niece while my sister took of her coat and got started on the evening meal. She was pregnant with her second child and already getting quite big.

'Anto, there is some paperwork for you to sign, on the dining table.'

I walked over to take a look at the papers. 'You know, Rose, I can't believe that you manage to juggle looking after Maria, working as a medic, looking after my affairs, keeping the house clean and cooking dinner. I cannot imagine how you do it. It takes all my energy to do one thing fairly well.' I knew there was a time when I could have done the same juggling act that my sister does, but I wasn't jealous. I admire her.

'Aunchie,' my niece called out.

'Yes, Maria,' I replied, returning to the sofa to sit next to her. 'Mmmm,' she continued, burying her face in my cheek for what seemed an eternity, her tiny arms embracing my neck. I turned and smiled at Rose.

'She rarely gives *me* a kiss like that,' smiled Rose. Was that a bit of admiration in my sister's voice?

Useful information

As my head injury was so long ago, some of the places I benefited from, such as Garston Manor, no longer exist. On the other hand, it does seem that there are many more resources now for people like me than there were a few years back, when we were forced to rely heavily on the private sector for rehabilitation.

Below are some organisations that have helped me a lot.

1. The Silverlining
A charitable organisation that provides a professionally supported environment for brain injury sufferers to make friendships and find meaning through interaction and helping others.
www.thesilverlining.org.uk

2. Headway
A charitable organisation that provides help and support for brain-injury sufferers and their families.
www.headway.org.uk

3. BIRT (part of The Disabilities Trust)
A charitable organisation that offers rehabilitation services, long-term housing and community care.
www.thedtgroup.org/brain-injury/

4. do-it!
National database of volunteering opportunities in the UK.
www.do-it.org.uk

The following is a short list of books that I and my family think are good.

Living with Brain Injury: A Guide for Families by Richard C. Senelick and Cathy E. Ryan (Partners Publishing Group, 2nd rev edn 1998).

Over My Head: A Doctor's Own Story of Head Injury from the Inside Looking Out by Claudia Osborn (Andrews McMeel, 2000).

Time out of Mind by Jane Lapotaire (Virago Press, new edn 2004).